Michelle Cree is a clinical psychologist who worked for seventeen years in the Derbyshire Perinatal Mental Health Service, where she pioneered the use of both individual- and compassion-focused therapy (CFT) for the perinatal population. She became a national and international trainer and supervisor in CFT and the compassionate mind approach, and is the author of *The Compassionate Mind Approach to Postnatal Depression: Using Compassion Focused Therapy to Enhance Mood, Confidence and Bonding*. This became the first perinatal mental health book to be selected for the Reading Well list (previously the Books on Prescription scheme).

Also by Michelle Cree

The Compassionate Mind Approach to Postnatal Depression: Using Compassion Focused Therapy to Enhance Mood, Confidence and Bonding

THE NEW MOTHERHOOD WORKBOOK

Developing a Compassionate Mind for
You, Your Baby and Your Family

MICHELLE CREE

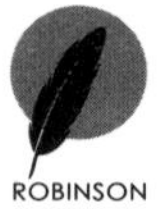

ROBINSON

ROBINSON

First published in Great Britain in 2025 by Robinson

1 3 5 7 9 10 8 6 4 2

Illustrations by Liane Payne

A CIP catalogue record for this book is available from the British Library.

ISBN: 978-1-47214-747-9

Typeset in Palatino by Initial Typesetting Services, Edinburgh
Printed and bound in Great Britain by Clays Ltd, Elcograf S.p.A.

Papers used by Robinson are from well-managed forests and other responsible sources.

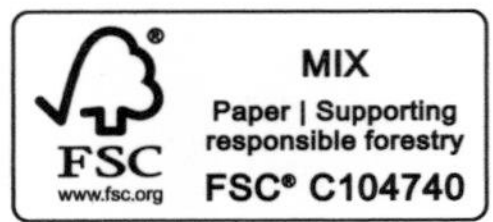

Robinson
An imprint of
Little, Brown Book Group
Carmelite House
50 Victoria Embankment
London EC4Y 0DZ

The authorised representative
in the EEA is
Hachette Ireland
8 Castlecourt Centre
Dublin 15, D15 XTP3, Ireland
(email: info@hbgi.ie)

An Hachette UK Company
www.hachette.co.uk

www.littlebrown.co.uk

*For Jacob, Thomas, Freya
and Neil*

Contents

Acknowledgements

I would like to thank my children and my husband for their encouragement, support and interesting ways of thinking about things. They are a collection of wonderful minds who have all contributed to making this book better.

I would like to express my heartfelt gratitude to Professor Paul Gilbert for bringing his astonishing mind to the enormous difficulty of how to alleviate and prevent suffering. His development of compassion-focused therapy and the compassionate mind approach has made such an immense impression on human suffering. It has been an honour and a privilege to be able to work with Paul to bring this approach to my particular field of mothers and babies.

I offer my gratitude also to the mothers I have worked with and encountered in my life, who all contributed such wisdom to this book. It is wonderful to be able to hand this wisdom on to other mothers and to their families.

In addition, I want to thank all those who make up my 'compassionate team' and enable me to do difficult things; including my family, friends and people I work with.

And thanks of course to Andrew McAleer and the team at Little, Brown for their work and support in bringing this book to fruition.

Foreword by Professor Paul Gilbert

It is ten years since I wrote a foreword for Michelle Cree's *The Compassionate Mind Approach to Postnatal Depression*. I am delighted to be able to do the same for this broader, updated workbook encompassing new motherhood more generally and providing a step-by-step approach with practical, interactive exercises.

In this book, Michelle breaks guidance down into a series of modules, exploring how evolution made our minds this way. None of us chose to have brains that could go into states of anxiety, panic, rage, depression and despair. We don't wake up in the morning and choose to experience these states or practise them! They come without our wishing or wanting them – hence they are not our fault and we need to exercise compassion with ourselves when we encounter them.

We have always understood that compassion is very important for our wellbeing. If we are stressed or upset it is always better to have kind, helpful and supportive people around us rather than critical, rejecting or disinterested folk. It is not only this common sense that tells us about the value of kindness and compassion; recent advances in scientific studies of compassion and kindness have greatly advanced our understanding of how these qualities really do influence and help us in all kinds of ways, both in body and mind. Yet we live in an age that can make compassion for ourselves and others difficult. This is the world of seeking the competitive edge, of achievement and desire, of comparison to others who are maybe doing better than us, and of dissatisfaction, self-disappointment and the tendency to be self-critical (sometimes very harshly). Research has now revealed that such environments actually make us unhappier, and that mental ill-health is on the increase, especially in younger people.

Having a baby can be a stressful time, when we need as much support and compassion from others as we can get. Medical care has progressed rapidly over the centuries and we now have a multitude of ways to facilitate the physical health of mother and baby. However, when it comes to psychological wellbeing, the story is somewhat different.

Mothers historically gave birth within integrated networks of relatives and friends. We are one of only a few primate species that pass our babies around and allow others to care for them from the first minutes of life. Importantly, we now know that not only does such support provide the mother with practical assistance but also that caring, social relationships have profound impacts on a range of physiological processes. There is now very good evidence that being a recipient of care impacts our cardiovascular, immune and hormonal systems, balances the autonomic nervous system and stimulates key neurocircuits in our brain. Being imbedded in caring relationships therefore impacts the psycho-physiological processes of birthing and post-birth adaptation, including how we relate to our baby.

However, we don't live in these communities in the same way today, and therefore it can be difficult for some mothers to feel supported in networks of female relatives and friends (who would be there to not only offer physical but also emotional help, advice and guidance). So it's important to recognise that, sometimes, through no fault of our own, we might not have the support that we ideally need. When we are struggling, we need to acknowledge this, without any shame, and reach out for help from health visitors or friends to share our feelings, even if they are ones of doubt, depression, confusion or anxiety.

Research has also shown that it is not just the care that we receive from others that can be crucial but also the relationships we have inside our own heads; the way we think and feel about ourselves. This is not difficult to appreciate. For example, imagine that you are struggling with something and people around you are critical or regard you as inadequate in some way. What do you think will happen in your brain and body; how will you feel? If, in contrast, there are people around you whom you trust, who are understanding and kind, and who you sense are keen to be helpful and supportive because they care about you, how is that going to feel in your brain and your body? Pretty obvious, really; it is going to feel very different, stimulate very different processes and help you feel that you will be able to cope and manage. So it is with our internal processes of self-criticism and compassion.

If we are struggling and we become harshly self-critical and view ourselves as inadequate or deficient in some way, we generate angry and hostile emotions towards ourselves and cause ourselves a lot of pain and suffering. It follows that, if we learn to be sensitive to our distress, and are empathic and understanding, then our brains and our bodies will respond quite differently. Keep in mind that, when we trigger compassion, we are also stimulating a number of physiological systems that can help us when we are distressed.

Michelle helps us understand why and how we can make compassion central to our way of being. She gently explores many of the complex issues around childbirth, the changes that take place in one's body that can produce unwanted mood changes or anxiety, and how they can sometimes turn off loving feelings. She also explores how we can get lost in loops of self-criticism through no fault of our own. And, most importantly, she shows how to reach out for help if we need it by dealing with things we might be ashamed of and learning how to treat ourselves more wisely and kindly.

Compassion can sometimes be viewed as being soft or weak – a way of letting our guard down and not trying hard enough. But actually, compassion enables us to be open to, and tolerant of, our painful feelings. Compassion is not about turning away from such emotional difficulties or discomforts, or trying to get rid of them, but instead it is about engaging with them and compassionately focusing on what is going to be helpful to flourish and take care of ourselves, enabling us to live our lives more fully and contentedly.

Michelle brings her many years of experience as a clinical psychologist, working with mothers-to-be and those who have had their baby – some with very major mental health difficulties or struggles with bonding to their baby. She also brings a wealth of experience from working with and training people in compassion-focused therapy for over twenty years. In this book, she outlines a model of compassion that seeks to stimulate and build your confidence in your own compassionate wisdom and strength, which will support you as you engage with the difficulties you may have.

This workbook helps you to develop compassionate motives, compassionate attention, compassionate feelings, compassionate thinking and compassionate behaviour. Michelle shows you step-by-step ways to become more mindful and aware of how your mind is working rather than being lost in the emotions that might be powerfully activated within you. Mindfulness helps us to notice but also to become more of an observer – we become aware that we are anxious or depressed, but we learn to be more observant of it rather than lost to it.

As Michelle indicates, taking the steps to be helpful to ourselves is not always easy because sometimes our emotions can have a real hold over us. Sometimes our emotions can be linked to negative feelings about ourselves, such as that we are in some way flawed, not able to be a good mother, or not as good as other mothers because of our struggles. Our threat systems can get control and texture our experience of life. This is why learning how to be mindful and to stand back and become more observant, rather than lost in some of our automatic processes, can be so helpful. In a way, it's like being in a fast-flowing river that's rushing you along but then you realise you can stand up, and when you do, you can see how the river is powerful but now flowing around you.

You will explore the potential power of working directly with your body by breathing in a particular way that helps to settle, ground and focus the body. You will discover practices for developing a kind voice within yourself and also using postures and facial expressions to stimulate systems in your brain and body.

Michelle guides you through a variety of compassionate thinking and imagery practices. These can be visual, auditory or sensory. For example, she shows you how to imagine a 'compassionate other' being compassionate to you, listening, understanding or even putting an arm around you. You can imagine their facial expression and kind, supportive voice tones. And you can sense their motivation to be helpful.

In fact, you already have intuitive wisdom on the essence of compassion. If you had a friend whom you really cared about and they were struggling with the same kinds of things you are struggling with, the chances are you would automatically try to be helpful and supportive rather than dismissive, blaming, hostile and critical. Consider how you would actually do that; how you would show your compassion for your friend and how they would experience that from you. This book builds on your own intuitive wisdom and how to apply it to yourself, despite any resistance you might have to doing that.

It is our motive to be helpful, not harmful, which is the basis of compassion; it is this orientation to life that can help us ride the waves of distress and find meaning and purpose. Michelle offers a wise and compassionate guide to the journey that seeks to support you in this phase of your life.

Professor Paul Gilbert PhD FBPsS OBE

November 2024

Introduction

This book might appear to be about a very specific and short time in a person's life; after all, it is a book about new motherhood. It covers the perinatal period, which is usually considered to be pregnancy, birth and the first one or two years of the baby's life. Yet it affects all of us. We have all been children. Most of us will have been 'mothered' in one way or another, and as with other important early relationships, we probably have a sense that we carry imprints from these with us into our adult life and then into our relationships with our children.

At first glance, using this workbook might seem an awful lot of effort to invest for this relatively small period of time – particularly when there is a lot to be going on with anyway. However, new mothers do buy books, go to classes, listen to podcasts, talk to lots of people, and spend a lot of time in one form or other trying to work out how to be the best parent they can.

Although these few months and years might seem a drop in the ocean compared to a lifetime, mothers spend so much time thinking about this because they know just what an impact mothering has, and what a disproportionate impact the early years have. And it is not just a huge amount of *thought* that mothers give over to this. Mothering involves so much of the body too. Pregnancy, giving birth, breastfeeding. But even if people become mothers without being pregnant, or never breastfeed, there is still so much of the body involved. Be it carrying the baby, offering the body as a protective 'home', facilitating the baby's exploration and the development of new skills, processing and regulating one's own emotions and those of the baby too. And so it goes on.

Despite this, mothering often seems to be the 'quiet' job, occurring in the background, without too much fuss, appreciation, value or understanding of just what a profound impact it has. It is not of course done for gratitude (although some helps) but instead aims to provide a steady ground from which children can springboard into the world. And like steady ground, it is not noticed until it gets shaky or crumbles altogether.

This book aims to provide a step-by-step guide to developing and maintaining a steady ground for mothers so that they can live lives of fulfilment and ease, whilst also providing a steady ground for their family, so that they can do the same.

The compassionate mind approach and compassion-focused therapy have been developed by clinical psychologist Professor Paul Gilbert as a culmination of his life's work into the science of what causes humans to suffer so much and what can be done to help to alleviate and prevent this suffering. And this, in part, is just what we do for our children: alleviate and prevent suffering by providing them with the skills of being able to live well, with ease, and to be able to be helpful to others.

It is focused specifically on the concept of compassion because we are wired as humans to be able to get through some very challenging and difficult aspects of our lives and to live well and flourish, when we experience the safeness that compassion gives us. Safeness can be in terms of a safe environment to live in, for example, but for humans our safeness comes primarily from our relationships. These might be our relationships with others, but also with ourselves. When we detect that people (or ourselves) are looking out for us, value us, and want to help and support us, then our body and mind operate in very different ways compared to when we feel unsafe and under threat. We become calmer, steadier, more able to take in the perspectives of others, more able to think, problem-solve, be creative, be playful and learn. We also become more courageous, confident and able to move out and engage with the world, with all its opportunities and challenges. This is just the same for our baby. And we don't even need a physical presence (although this helps). Drawing on memories and the knowledge that we are supported works too.

As parents, our compassionate mind also creates a particular pattern in our mind and body that enables us to best understand the mind of our child, and be able to attune to them and interact with them in a skilful and sensitive manner. This creates the bedrock of a secure attachment and their own compassionate mind, so that they in turn can go out into the world with as much steadiness, helpfulness and ability to make their own positive relationships as possible.

So, this book has a double impact, on our own mind and body but also on the mind and body of our baby too. This then spreads out like waves to other members of our family and people whom we, and our family, then encounter.

Such a lot can come from those tiny, quiet moments that can seem so inconsequential, between us and our baby, us and others, but also us and our own mind.

How the book works

Each section of this book builds on the previous one, so it is designed to be done step by step, preferably in order. Inevitably, you might be drawn to a particular section and might end up jumping about, but as long as the book is working for you, it doesn't really matter how you approach it.

It is designed to be interactive so that you can think in much more depth about each aspect. It will prompt you to think about yourself, your baby, and also your partner, because there are likely to be other people in your life who are parenting with you.

Hopefully, this will be a fascinating, enjoyable and helpful process for you, and for your baby and family.

Section 1:
Preparing the ground for our compassionate mind

Module 1: Using this workbook

This is a workbook, so it is different to reading a normal book. It is a book for you to interact with and work through, step by step. It is your book so you can make it your own. It should be a book which you feel comfortable with and enjoy interacting with.

You might be somebody who likes to keep a book pristine, or someone who folds down corners, or uses a beautiful bookmark or an old chocolate wrapper to mark where you are. You might want to underline important bits, write in the margins, and fill in the sections in the book. Or perhaps you would rather have a separate book or folder to fill out and keep this one unmarked. You can also download resources from https://overcoming.co.uk/715/resources-to-download so that you can keep them wherever you wish. You may not enjoy writing, or find it difficult, so perhaps you might prefer to record your answers or talk them into a writing app that can write them down for you.

However you decide to do it, the aim of this book is to really deepen your learning about yourself, and the process of you becoming a mother to your baby. Having a baby is a very sensory experience, and babies learn through all their senses and from interacting with the world in a very curious and playful way. We will be learning a lot from our baby, so we can bring how they learn to this book too. Sometimes it is hard to be playful, especially if that is not our nature. Perhaps we never really learned how to play, or life may feel too serious at the moment to be playful. But feeling a little more at ease helps us to shift our brain into a state where learning, and also compassion, come a bit easier. It can unlock us from the constraints that our threat brain necessarily puts us in, and can open up a whole lot of sometimes surprising and helpful possibilities.

As you will come to see later in this book, our breath is an amazing portal into different mental and physical states, and it is always with us. It is a wonderful way in to feeling a little looser and calmer. So just start with breathing in and letting your breath come out slowly, as if enjoying breathing in some fresh countryside air. Do this as many times as you wish.

Now move and stretch your arms and legs as if you are limbering and loosening up to start a jog or an exercise session.

In the box below (or you may wish to put all of the following in your own notebook, journal or folder) write something like: 'This is my book and I'm going to write in it' or 'Hello book!' or whatever you would like to write to start off your interaction with it. Write it in pen, pencil, crayon, paint, different colours – whatever you like:

In this box, stick a picture or postcard or anything that you would really enjoy looking at when you open your book:

In this box, do a drawing or make some marks with your baby, or as if from your baby, as they are part of this journey with you too (even if they are not yet here or are no longer here):

This box is for sticking or drawing anything that reminds you of people who are important in your journey of becoming a mother. Perhaps your partner, a family member, or somebody else from the past. This reminds us that we are never parenting alone, even if the person is someone we carry in our memory:

In this box, if you can, add something that reminds you of a smell that you like. Alternatively, write down or stick in a picture of what it is:

In this box, if you can, add a texture that feels nice to you, perhaps a piece of fabric, a little bit of fur from your dog or cat, an especially smooth piece of paper. Or write down what the texture would be, or stick in a picture of it, and see if it is possible to keep something that reminds you of the texture with this book:

Write in this box sounds that you like to hear – perhaps birdsong, a baby's giggle, a cat's purr, your mum's humming, or maybe a certain song or instrument. You might be able to record the sounds on your phone, perhaps making a library of things that you can listen to when you wish:

My notes and reflections on this section (for example, what you want to hold onto and remember, or make a note to do):

At the back of the book is a section where you can add notes that you want to remember as you go through the book so that you can build up your own list of what you have found helpful. You can also download resources from https://overcoming.co.uk/715/resources-to-download to add to your own notebook or journal.

Module 2: My motivational systems

We come to motherhood, not as a blank slate, but with experiences that have shaped us, a brain and body shaped by evolution, and a set of genes that we didn't choose. These, along with many other factors such as the people around us, and the environment and the culture we live in, will have a profound effect on us as mothers; how we experience motherhood, and how we mother. We are only just scratching the surface of all the different factors, both inside of us and outside of us, that come together to influence becoming a mother.

However, all these different influences are not just done *to* us, leaving us helpless as to the outcome. Science is also helping us to understand just what we can influence. We can imagine our minds as like a garden, tended and grown for us by evolution, genes and our experiences growing up, in a way which is largely out of our control. However, we now know that we can step into that garden and take control of how we want it to be. We cannot transform it totally. We can't make it a hot and dry garden if it is in a cool and rainy place for example, but we can work on areas of it, bringing in good compost, weeding it, tending to it and watering it. With our more recent understandings of neuroplasticity (that we can continue learning and changing our brain for our whole lives) and of epigenetics (that we can actually turn genes on and off), we no longer need to feel that the brain, body, genes and experiences (particularly early ones) are our lot. We now know that we can work on developing a slightly different version of ourselves and live our lives in a different way to the way we have done so far. What version of yourself would you choose to work towards?

We have evolved to have a number of systems to help us do the tasks of living. For example, we have three basic motivational systems: one concerned with keeping us safe from threat, another that drives us to go and get the resources (such as food, protection and shelter) needed for ourselves and our children to survive, and a third that motivates us to rest, digest, recuperate and heal. We also have more social motivational systems; for example, those that drive us to be seen positively by other people, so they are more likely to help us when we need it, those for competing with others (for example, to get those important resources), and those that are about caring for others and being cared for. We don't choose these, but they are part of us because they have been so crucial in the survival of our species. They will be guiding and driving us, and our baby, to a greater or lesser extent, probably every day.

We now have a much clearer understanding of what helps us to function well, and indeed to flourish as human beings, but particularly so when we have a baby. These are the same aspects that then help to shape and tend the 'garden' of our baby's mind so that they can best function and flourish in life too. These aspects focus on the particular response humans have to safeness and connection, particularly in relationships. And this applies whether we are offering, or receiving, that safeness and connection, or indeed if we are giving this to ourselves.

This has been called our 'compassionate mind' by Paul Gilbert, a professor of clinical psychology who has spent his working life investigating scientifically and clinically what best helps us, especially when we are suffering. He has particularly focused on those who have experienced high levels of shame and self-criticism and as a result were experiencing severe depression and anxiety. The model he has developed is, at its heart, the science of how humans best flourish and has now been applied to just about every human experience that you can imagine. So, this book focuses on the particular motivational system of caring for others and being cared for, but also more specifically in order to prevent and alleviate suffering – the motivational system of compassion. Hopefully, we will see that it can be very powerfully applied to the process and experience of motherhood, especially when we are having a difficult time or need to find courage or build our confidence: not just for mothers, parents, siblings and the wider family, but for our baby too.

This book will take us step by step through this process of developing our compassionate mind as a mother, and of developing the compassionate mind of our baby too (and hopefully catching all sorts of other people up in the process as well!).

What brought you to this book?

There was something that meant you are now holding this book and beginning to look through it. What was it?

What brought you to this book?

____

____

____

What are your hopes for this book?

Sometimes we come to things because of the fear of negatives; for example, 'I don't want to be the kind of parent that my mother was' or 'I don't want to get depressed' or 'I don't want my baby to turn out like me'. We naturally do this because, as we will see, our threat system often has the loudest voice. This is not our fault; it is just what has been shaped in humans to help us survive. However, it means that we end up only having an image of how we don't want to be, not how we do want to be.

So, what would you see if the book did what you hoped it would? (Be as specific as possible, describing what you would see as if you had filmed it on your phone, e.g. the manner in which you were interacting with a particular person, the way you speak and sound, new activities you might be trying and the manner in which you would be doing them, etc.)

What would your partner see if the book had helped you in the way you hoped? (Again, describe it as if you were watching a film clip of it.)

What would your baby see and experience if the book had done what you hoped it would?

Visualising our hopes, as clearly and concretely as possible, helps to give us an image of what we are heading towards, like putting a flag on a distant mountain. It is then easier to notice when we are moving in that direction. It is quite different to taping off areas that we don't want to go into, because then our attention is focused backwards and only on the negatives – on not ending up where we don't want to go, and looking at how close or far we are from the 'no-go' areas, without a clear direction that we actually want to travel in. This book will be about getting greater and greater clarity about where we are heading, whilst guiding us towards it and then helping us to make it our place when we get there. The compassionate mind journey though is a life's work. As we will see, our threat mind is designed to forever be pulling us into patterns we don't want. This is just how it is, no matter how practised we are with our compassionate mind. But we can learn how to shift into a much better place, more and more quickly each time, creating a way of life and of being, rather than a set of techniques we use only when we remember. This book will hopefully help us to shift a few degrees onto a different course which over time will make a bigger and bigger difference to us and the people around us. It is about building the life we want and helping us to maintain it. But it will be step by step, no rush – we have our whole life to be working on and practising this. It will just get easier and easier over time, like rolling a snowball down a hill.

As humans, we often set off with good intentions but then find it hard or get disillusioned when we don't get the results we hoped for or as quickly as we hoped. This may well happen with this book.

What has helped you commit to things for the long run, even when things got hard? (For example, sticking at school, learning to drive, completing a training course, completing a difficult task, becoming and sticking with being a parent, facing something that scares you but is important to you to face.)

____

____

____

What will help you get back on track if you give up on the book for a bit? What will help you to remember why this is important to you? What will help remind you of what you have inside you already that helps you do difficult things? (Perhaps it is just something you write down and put with your phone, or a photo or picture or object that represents your qualities and where you are wanting to head.)

____

____

____

My reflections and notes on this section (what you want to hold on to and remember, or points you want to take forward to work on, for example).

____

____

____

____

____

____

Module 3: Why a 'compassionate mind'?

Wishes for our baby

If one of those wise old women from a fairy story appeared at the birth of your child and said, 'to celebrate the birth of this new person in the world, I will grant you three wishes for your child', what would your wishes be?

Your wishes for your child

____

____

____

____

____

____

Our wishes for our children often follow particular themes: to be happy, to be well and healthy, to be confident, to have enough money to feel safe, secure and unworried, to have good friends, to bring a little bit of good to the world, to be able to get through and bounce back from any difficulties that life throws at them.

It is not usually things like 'to keep everyone at a distance, to be wealthy at all costs, to be harmful to others and to go through life being disruptive and annoying'.

Intuitively we know that there is a pattern or way of being that is particularly beneficial for us as human beings. Something about confidence, steadiness, joyfulness, the ability to be part of a group that supports us and that we can in return support as best we can, as well as a strength that allows us to get back up after the knocks of life.

What kind of parents are you hoping to be?

Imagine you are a grand old age and looking back over your life. Write down here a quick description of the kind of mother you would be glad to see that you had been.

____

____

____

____

____

Hazarding a guess, you might have listed something like warm, kind, encouraging, wise and supportive. Someone who had the courage to stand up and fight for your child if necessary and the strength to help them through difficult times. Someone with the ability to guide them, teaching them the skills and encouraging the qualities that help them both to flourish and to get through, and bounce back from, the inevitable difficulties of life.

If this is so, then what we are talking about here is what might be called 'the compassionate mind'. Paul Gilbert defined this as a mind that:

'is sensitive to suffering and has a commitment to alleviating and preventing that suffering in ourselves and others',

In other words, a mind that wishes to be

'helpful and not harmful'

and that

'takes joy from seeing oneself and others flourish'

As we will see, this kind of mind brings a whole wealth of advantages to us mentally, to how we think, but also to our body. It is also a mind that brings something very important to parenting and, in turn, helps our children to develop their own compassionate mind.

Now, of course, we could all have ideals about how we would like to be and what we would like to become, but most of the time we fall rather short of them. An ideal gives us a direction, but what is also important is how we treat ourselves and others when it doesn't go to plan. For many of us, when we are disappointed in ourselves, we become cross, self-critical and sometimes quite harsh with ourselves. Even when we do well, we still might brush this off and put ourselves down for feeling a little bit pleased. This is where compassion comes in, because compassion is there to support us in times of disappointment, upset, setback and struggle. As the definition says, it's about how we deal with suffering. It is also there to take joy in ourselves and be pleased when things do go well.

What kind of mother/father do you think your partner would wish to have been when they look back?

___

___

___

By bringing our 'ideal future selves' to mind with as much detail as possible, it helps us to bring clarity and focus to what is important to us, and we are then much more likely to make it happen. It gives us a clear and conscious aim; even if we have ups and downs (one thing we can be sure of), overall, this is what we are working towards.

What aspects of you and your parenting would you like your baby to take into their parenting if they had a baby?

___

___

___

What aspects of your partner would you hope your baby would take into themselves if your baby became a parent?

___

As our baby grows, our mind is wired to take more notice of the bad than the good. It is what kept us safe. However, it is not great for our self-compassion or the sense of ourselves as even a half-decent parent. These exercises are therefore helpful to come back to over time in order to shift our focus to the aspects that are actually going well in the moment, and to remind ourselves of how these moments are building the future for ourselves and our child too.

This is the same with our parents or parental figures. We may think there is nothing whatsoever that we would want to take with us from them into our parenting. And perhaps, tragically, that is the case. However, for all but the most horrifying of parents there is usually at least one aspect of them that people would take with them, in some form or other. Rarely is it the case that people would throw away every aspect of a parent. Often these more positive aspects appear over time, particularly as we go through the parenting journey ourselves, and start to look at our own parents with different eyes.

The same for our children. In order to do the hard job of separating from us, they have to 'rubbish' us – sometimes even our very breathing or presence becomes annoying to them. This is an evolved drive, not one they have chosen to possess, which helps our children with the task of having to grow up and leave us after their lifetime (to that point) of being wired to stay close to us. Once they have done this, they can settle into their adult selves. As their security in this grows, they can begin to take back the parts of us and their childhood that they want to bring to their own children. This is a long wait when you are a new parent. But it can help to hold in mind that the good bits that we do on the way are being taken in by our children, like nuts stored by squirrels, to be taken out in years to come, even if our child doesn't consciously realise that we put them there.

What is so good about this 'compassionate mind'?

Imagine you have a baby who is very unsettled and only sleeps for short periods of time (perhaps it's not so hard to imagine for you). You contact the health visiting team for some help. The health visitor arrives. Her name is Janine. She seems a little short-tempered and annoyed. She gives you some advice that you've already tried and seems a bit cross when you say so. She tells you that you need to try it again and this time commit to it properly. She gives you a leaflet and hurries off. She is clearly very busy.

How might you be left feeling?

Instead of Janine (she is far too busy to come), Sheila arrives. Sheila seems warm and kind. She listens carefully and seems to understand just how hard this has been for you. She asks about what you have tried and how it went. She asks about what milk your baby has, what you are eating if you are breastfeeding, how your pregnancy was, what happened during labour and delivery, and how you are recovering. She asks about the support you are getting and also checks your baby over. She suggests a variety of things that she can try with you but gives you a plan of what to try first. She says that she will ring you in a few days to see how you have got on, and also arranges a time to come and see you again in a week.

How might you be left feeling?

You might be thinking here, 'Well of course I'd feel better with Sheila rather than Janine. This is not really telling me anything new.' It might seem so obvious that we dismiss it without really thinking about it. But when we dig into it, we start to uncover some important differences that demonstrate what helps and what hinders us functioning at our best as humans. We will also see that these differences require particular skills and attributes, as well as the right circumstances, to be able to behave as Sheila did. It is not necessarily as easy as we might think.

So why might a struggling mum feel better with Sheila than Janine?

From the moment we open the door to either health visitor, a whole cascade of brain and body responses occurs. The impact of either Janine or Sheila's visit could be considerable and potentially more long-lasting than we might expect. And as we will see, this can particularly be the case during this unique perinatal period, because we have evolved to need the help of others at this time, even more than we normally do. Encountering unhelpful people at this time can make us feel vulnerable, which can be quite disconcerting, particularly if this kind of thing wouldn't normally wobble us.

We are going to look in detail at some of the many responses that take place in interactions with others (and with ourselves) in order to give us clarity about how to consciously develop our own compassionate mind and that of our baby. It will also help to develop our understanding of what happens when we feel more under threat or more safe.

My reflections and notes on this section (what you want to hold onto and remember, or points you want to take forward to work on, for example).

Section 2:

Developing the skills of our compassionate mind

Module 4: Old brain, new brain

Areas within our old brain are largely concerned with the functions that we share with many other animals, such as guarding territory, finding food, reproducing, fleeing or attacking predators.

We may describe some of these a little differently in humans but they are still powerful motivational systems within us. We have a very strong 'fight or flight' system which we experience as anger and anxiety. When we are hungry our mind gets focused on thinking about and finding food, no matter how annoying and inconvenient this might be. When we reach adolescence, suddenly we start all sorts of behaviour that may never have interested us before in terms of finding a mate. And we only need to think about how we might like to sit in the same place at home or work, or watch our children fight to keep others off 'their' piece of play equipment in the park, to see how territorial we still are. We have this strong tendency to defend what is ours, or protect the space that we find safe, because these strategies have served us well in our very ancient past, but also still potentially serve us well now. These strategies get passed on in our genes – in the past, those who defended their territory or their possessions were more likely to survive than those who didn't.

So, our potentially very possessive and territorial nature, our urges to fight or flee, our motivation to find food or a mate, are not our fault. These have in effect been selected for us by nature, rather than by us. When we have a baby, we might notice these feelings feel even stronger than before. We are going to see just how much our urges and motivational systems are not our fault. As this unfolds, this can help us to take a different position towards ourselves. Rather than perhaps attacking ourselves for these urges or being confused by them, we can begin to accept that these are part of our nature as humans. Then we can also work with them and try to guide and shape these urges or motivational systems if we wish.

What old brain activities have you done so far today?

____

____

____

Old brain: Care-giving and care-receiving

Still considered part of the 'old brain' but much newer in evolutionary terms are motivational systems to do with looking after offspring and being looked after. We can think about these as the motivational systems that we might share with our dog, for example.

Imagine a day in the life of a pet dog. What might it get up to?

____

____

____

Thinking about a dog's life; they like to guard their territory, be fed, reproduce, be with their owner, be patted, stroked and played with. And when they have puppies, they stay close and care for them. So, as well as all these evolutionarily ancient systems, such as protecting our territory and so on, now we have these newer systems which we share with our dog, of wanting to care for our offspring, wanting to be cared for, wanting closeness, affection and playfulness. The attachment system, which is where a baby has systems designed to keep it close to its parents, and the bonding system, which is where parents have systems designed to keep their baby close to them, are part of this care-giving, care-receiving motivational system. Compare this to reptiles where there is mainly short-lived caring (for example, crocodiles carry their babies tenderly in their mouths and keep them close for a few months to a year or more), or no caring at all, like we see in turtles who lay their eggs in holes dug in the sand. When their babies hatch, the mothers are nowhere to be seen. The babies must rely on their instincts to survive all the predators waiting for them. There is no mother to protect them, get food for them or teach them skills.

With mammals, there is this evolved motivational system of wanting to look after our offspring, keep them close, teach them skills, and so on. And our offspring have a motivational system that fits this like a key fits a lock. So, they have a system that wants to be physically close, that gets upset if they are not, that wants to be cared for and wants to learn new skills. We will see that it isn't necessarily as straightforward as this for the baby or the parent, and that, particularly in humans, all sorts of factors come into play with this process, such as our upbringing, our experiences and our genes. Like other mammals, the human motivational system to be maternal towards our offspring can be turned down or interrupted by many factors, which we will look at later in the book.

Returning to the day in the life of our dog, we also see the urge to play and be sociable. On the nature programmes we can witness this real drive amongst bear or fox cubs to play with each other, developing important life skills including how to interact with each other and how far to go with the physical rough and tumble.

How have you seen these motivations for care-giving, care-receiving, being playful, and for socially relating play in your baby today (e.g. play, wanting to be cared for, being caring of others when older, using you as a 'secure base' when they want to go out and explore, using you as a 'safe haven' when they get upset and want comfort, or need calming down if things get too much for them)?

____

____

____

How have your motivational systems for care-giving, care-receiving, being playful, and wanting to connect to others been showing up today (e.g. caring for baby, wanting to be cared for, playing with your baby, awareness of concern for others, wanting to connect with people, or struggling to connect)?

____

____

____

When we have a baby, and even during pregnancy, we can develop a strong bond with our baby, find it hard to leave them, feel physically calmer when we hold them, feel protective of them, even aggressively so. As already mentioned, this is not necessarily the case for many mothers – these feelings may take a while to appear because of factors such as a difficult birth, exhaustion, lack of support, chronic severe stress, depression, anxiety, or an ill baby. We will look at this in more detail later in the book. But it's not just our baby and children who want to be cared for. In fact, this need to feel safe and cared for never leaves us, no matter how independent and 'grown-up' we become. It is actually a really important system that helps us to function at our best in many different ways, as we shall see.

Have you noticed any changes in wanting to be cared for in yourself since becoming pregnant and having your baby? If so, what changes have you noticed?

____

____

____

Mothers and others with regard to care-giving and care-receiving

In perinatal terms, it seems that our need to be cared for may be turned up more when we become pregnant and have a baby, whether we want that to happen or not. This is because, if we look back through our history, for a large part of our time as early humans, we were living a potentially hazardous life; for example, on the African plains. There would have been attacks from other groups, difficulty in getting food whilst carrying and feeding a baby, and many predators that would particularly focus on targeting our defenceless baby as potentially easy prey.

We can see just how vulnerable we would be when we were pregnant, or breastfeeding, or carrying our baby or child. We would have become much more reliant on the care and help from others during this time including when we were giving birth. (Because of the way the human pelvis and birth canal have developed, mothers and their baby are much more likely to survive if we have assistance during childbirth.) We see that we are one of the few species in the animal kingdom who share the care of their offspring with others, and that when that care is available (for example, from grandmothers or partners), then the baby is much more likely to survive, and the mother is more able to sensitively interact with her baby.

This dependence on others would have led to us having a particularly increased vigilance as to how we were held in the minds of others during this perinatal time; 'Do they like me? Will they help me? Have I upset somebody? Would they be more likely to help me or that other mother with her baby if our group was in danger? Do they care about my child?'

This heightened attention to our social relationships during the perinatal period is likely to have been passed on through our genes. Those attending to social relationships are more likely to survive, as are their offspring. This means that our focus on being held positively in the minds of others to an even greater degree during the perinatal time is still a strong motivational system within us today, even if we are living in a society where we may be able to bring up our baby on our own with little help.

For those who have learned not to rely on others, finding that our brain and body seems to be doing its own thing during pregnancy and postnatally can be confusing and potentially difficult. For example, anecdotally many women report having a strong wish to have their mothers with them during and after birth. They describe it as being like an evolutionary urge that gets awakened during pregnancy and postnatally, even if their own mother is someone they have a difficult relationship with, they have broken contact with, or who may have died. This can create a great deal of painful and confusing feelings but might reflect our evolved wiring to be looked after and to have help at this critical time. Indeed, this fits with the evidence that the involvement of the grandmother increases the survival chances of both the mother and her baby: in humans, but also in other species too. On an individual basis our personal experience might not fit with this, but nevertheless the urge for an ideal mother might.

These motivational systems of care-giving and care-receiving are therefore really ramped up when we become pregnant and have our baby. We will see later in the book, just how complex this system or 'ramping up' is, how this might not be the case for everyone, and how none of this is our fault.

Our baby is born with a system to attach and be cared for, which is vital for its survival. And it is not long before we see that our baby also appears to be wired to be caring towards others too, even from quite a young age.

These particular motivational systems of wanting to care for and being cared for form the foundation of our compassion motivation. But compassion requires abilities that sit in the new brain, not just these old brain motivations of caring and being cared for. So, what does the 'new brain' do?

New brain

We've looked at our 'old brain', so what about our 'new brain'? This is the lumpy, folded outside part that we see when we look at a whole human brain. There are many different ways in which we can think about the different, amazing competencies of our human brain compared to other animals. Compassion-focused therapy suggests three basic competencies, but there are others.

Firstly, we have a capacity for understanding how systems work and for reasoning. We call this the scientific mind – the mind that can problem-solve. Think how much we problem-solve through everyday life, working out how to juggle the needs of our baby with the needs of others, how to get to a new place, how to work our new phone. We can also reason about ourselves, and this is called metacognition. We can have judgements as to whether we're doing well or not so well; we can imagine ourselves in the future in good places or not such good places. So we can look forward to things and make plans for the future but also worry and ruminate. As far as we know, no other animal can do this.

The second skill is a kind of empathy – the ability to tune in and understand that we and other people do the things we do because we have motives and emotions. One of the things that's important in being a mother is how we are able to empathise with our baby. We try to work out if they're crying because they need to feed or because they're cold or because of their colic. Empathic reasoning is reasoning about the nature of minds, and humans are much better at it than any other animal. Sometimes we get it wrong, though, and we make assumptions about what other people or babies are thinking or feeling when it's not the case.

The third function is our ability to be self-aware and to be aware that we have thoughts and feelings; we can pay attention to our thoughts as they arise but we can also judge them and become self-conscious and self-critical. We can knowingly and deliberately pay attention to things around us. We can deliberately choose to focus on enjoying a summer's day or the taste of certain food. We can also understand that our minds might be too threat-focused and that we would like to learn different ways of becoming calmer and steadier, perhaps by working through this book. As far as we are aware, a lion or cat is unable to be aware of any necessary self-improvements and then to deliberately choose to undertake them, such as mindfulness lessons or some weight-training to help their hunting skills.

As we will see later in the book, these three competencies are wonderfully useful but, like all of our human psychology, they can also be harmful and cause suffering to others and to ourselves if used in certain ways.

So, the new brain is what gives us our incredible ability to imagine, to wonder about the future, to think, to problem-solve, to communicate by writing or painting or making a sculpture, and to understand what might be going on in the mind of another person. This 'new brain' is so well developed in humans that we have learned to work together in order to be able to live in almost any terrain on earth, in incredibly complex social groups, and have even managed to get ourselves off our planet.

However, this new brain that helps us to do such incredible things can also be a source of immense suffering for us. Because we have both an 'old brain' and a 'new brain', they can fire each other off in what can be really unhelpful ways. For example, when we have our baby, we can look into the future and worry about them becoming ill, or us becoming ill. Our 'old brain', which is on the lookout for survival threat and safeness, then gets stimulated by this new brain thought, which triggers off a whole suite of responses to do with anxiety. The more anxious our 'old brain' makes us feel, the more our 'new brain' can spiral down into 'what if' catastrophic thoughts.

Paul Gilbert calls this 'the tricky brain' where the old brain and new brain get caught in these loops.

As far as we know, when a dog has puppies, she isn't worrying that one day they might get ill, whether she is going to be a good parent, or how quickly she is losing her baby weight. It is only because we have this set-up with both the 'old' and the 'new' brain that we can uniquely suffer in this way. And this is not our fault.

What loops might your baby's brain have got into if they had your new brain attached to their old brain?

____

____

____

Getting out of these old brain new brain loops

What loops have you found your brain to have got into recently?

____

____

____

____

____

If you can't think of any, perhaps use an example like this: you feel anxiety in your body ('old brain'). You are not sure why. You start searching around in your mind for why you might be anxious, worried you might have missed something important that you are supposed to be worrying about ('new brain'). This further stimulates your old brain to produce anxiety symptoms. You then respond to your increased anxiety by thinking there really must be something serious that you are supposed to be worrying about – and so on.

Another example is feeling you've said something silly ('new brain') which creates a feeling of anxiety, making your face flush red ('old brain'). You then become even more self-conscious of your red face ('new brain'), which drives the anxiety of your old brain, making you go even more red.

Imagine that you can sit watching this interaction going on between your old and new brain, but you are watching with a critical mind. What might you be saying in your mind?

____

____

____

What might the impact of this be?

____

____

____

How is it making you feel?

____

____

____

What is happening in your body? If the feelings and sensations in your body were to grow and grow – what is the urge in your body?

____

____

____

Now imagine watching this interaction, but without any judgement, just watching with curiosity (this is mindfulness) – how might this feel?

____

____

____

What might you be saying in your mind (if anything)?

____

____

____

What is your body wanting to do? If this feeling were to grow and grow in your body, what would the urge be in your body? What would your body want to do if you let it?

____

____

____

This second example – of choosing on purpose to attend to something in a manner which is non-judgemental – is the definition of mindful attention. This type of attention removes rather than adds to the fuel that keeps the loops going. We might notice that we begin to calm down.

The old brain no longer feels under attack and the new brain is now becoming more reflective. We can bring this mindful attention not just to our mind and our thoughts but also to sounds, tastes, any senses in fact, as well as to body sensations, even to pain in our body. We will be looking at mindfulness in more detail later in the book and will be exploring some of these different mindfulness practices.

This state of mindful awareness is similar to the state we might see in our baby and which is sometimes referred to as 'quiet alert' (we will be looking at the different physiological and emotional states of our baby later). It is the state our baby is in when we are carrying them and they are just looking around, taking in the world around them in a calm, curious manner. It is the best state for learning new information. It is also a state of steadiness and stability. This state is going to be one we come back to later when we look in more detail about how we can use our body to help create a mind which helps us to learn, but which is also the basis of courage, of being able to do difficult things, from a position of strength rather than fear or aggression.

Mindfulness is an incredibly powerful tool, and is even being taught in schools to children who are finding that they feel less angry and anxious, and calmer and better able to regulate their emotions.

Now imagine watching this interaction between your old and new brain with real kindness and understanding, with a real wish to be of help to this mother with her new baby (you), caught unintentionally in this loop. Imagine a warm, kind face and tone of voice talking to her (you). What might it say?

____

____

____

How does this make you feel if you imagine hearing this?

What thoughts might be running through your mind?

What is your body wanting to do? If the feelings in your body were to grow and grow, what is the urge in your body?

Did you notice a difference between the second exercise (mindfulness) compared to this one? In this one we are bringing in additional signals to ourselves of warmth, kindness and compassion. We react to this just as we would react to someone else who is being kind, warm and caring to us. It makes us feel safe. When we feel safe, our brain and body get organised into a particular pattern where we might feel calmer, can think more easily and more creatively, where we feel more accepted and connected to other people rather than disconnected, more confident and courageous. It is very powerful.

However, you might have noticed a resistance in you to the compassionate exercise. We can feel uncomfortable with compassion for all sorts of reasons. It might feel so uncomfortable or difficult that you want to avoid it. We will look later in the book at fears, blocks and resistances that people might have to any of the three flows of compassion; compassion to others, compassion from others to ourselves, and self-compassion.

Here is another example demonstrating how to get out of these tricky loops between our old and new brain.

Imagine that your baby has got upset whilst you are pushing them round a busy park in their buggy. Your new brain begins to worry that other people are getting cross that your baby is disturbing the peace. The more you worry, the more your old brain feels there is some kind of danger and makes your heart beat faster. Your old brain directs your attention to the faces of the people around you, scanning for annoyance. Your baby senses your agitation and gets more agitated themselves.

Firstly, imagine that you are looking down from a cloud just observing this process, with a curious, accepting, non-judgemental mind.

How do you feel now?

____

____

Rate how you are feeling from 0 to 10 (where 0 is calm, settled, and 10 is as awful as you can feel).

____

Secondly, imagine that you look down from the cloud with a wise, warm, kind, understanding mind, which wants to be as helpful as it can.

How do you feel now?

____

____

Rate how you are feeling from 0 to 10 (where 0 is calm, settled, and 10 is as awful as you can feel).

____

Hopefully, you have found that stepping outside of the loops and observing in a mindful way slows down and perhaps even stops the spiral into anxiety and criticism.

When we add compassion to mindfulness it can have even more power, as we are now feeling safe.

When our old brain and new brain drive each other in these loops it can be very difficult to stop it, or even to notice that it is happening. It is like we have fallen in a river and are being carried along helplessly by the current. But what if we could get out of the river and sit on the bank, watching the process rather than being in it? This is where the wonder of our new brain comes in. As humans we can use it to help us out of these loops and potential downward spirals. It has the ability to allow us to deliberately observe our own mind and body. And, to choose the manner in which we observe it. We could watch these loops with a critical mind; 'What a complete mess you get yourself into. Nobody else gets in such a state!' Or as we've seen, we could watch these loops with a compassionate mind; 'How hard is this to have both an old brain and a new brain, neither of which we chose but which can interact with each other and cause us to suffer so much.'

Our baby doesn't have such a well-developed new brain yet, so they are wonderfully unself-conscious. They don't worry about spitting out their food in a cafe, sticking a finger up Granny's nose, staring hard at the odd-looking man in the shop, or howling at the top of their lungs in the supermarket trolley. They are much more 'old brain', and 'in the moment' rather than looking forwards or backwards, or ruminating or worrying about the future. Our baby can really help us to see the impact that the development of our new brain abilities has on us as we grow up; that so much of what we come to struggle with is really not our fault, but just the way nature, and our experiences, many of which we did not choose, have come to shape us.

Odd as it might sound, sometimes a helpful way of bringing compassion to ourselves is to imagine how our dog, or a friend's dog, might react to a situation. We could have been born a dog, without this new brain, and life would have been much simpler; no self-criticism, no worrying about the future, no critical comparisons to others (although perhaps a dog has its own troubles where a new brain might have been helpful, like understanding that its owner will be back later). But we are human, with our particular brain set-up, which we are coming to learn about and manage as best we can, and as well as causing us some unique problems, it also brings some amazing aspects to our lives.

Your reflections and notes on this module about the old brain/new brain and getting out of its tricky loops.

What do you want to hold onto and remember? What would you like to take forward from here?

____

____

____

____

____

____

Module 5: The three circles: Our three emotion regulation systems

We've been talking about the different systems within us quite a lot, particularly the threat system. So, what do we mean by these different systems?

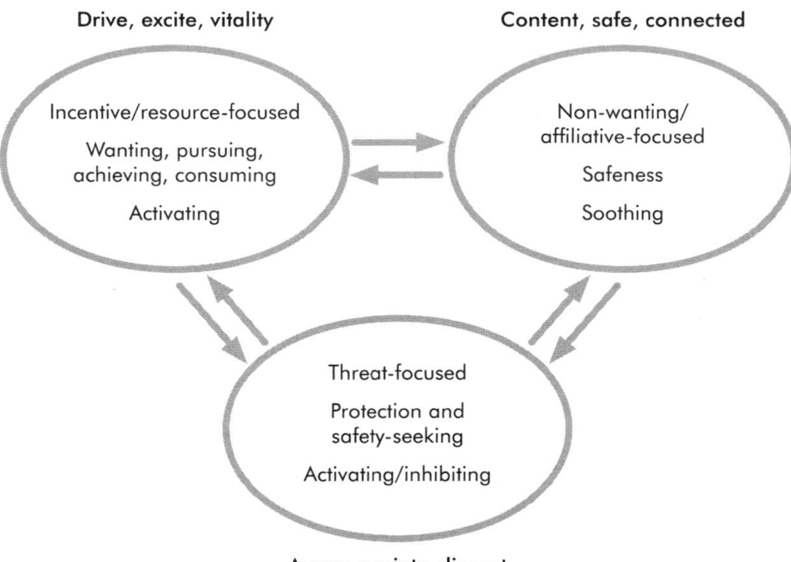

Figure 1: The Three Circles – Reproduced with permission from Gilbert, *The Compassionate Mind* (Robinson 2009)

These are often referred to as 'the three circles' in compassionate mind work. They represent three key motivational systems within us (and actually within many animals).

Types of emotion and emotion regulation

Compassion-focused therapy highlights the fact that all living things have three basic life tasks. Firstly, all living things must detect threats and possible harms to their existence and have some way of dealing with them. For example, trees will curl their leaves with a shortage of water, the bacteria in our gut will move away from areas which are toxic to them. So, because one of the main life tasks is identifying and dealing with threat, we also need emotions to prepare our body to take appropriate action. Different types of threat require a different type of response, so under some threats we might become angry while under others we might become anxious or run away. If the threat is to do with food that looks as if it's gone off, then we might have the emotion of disgust to keep us from eating it.

We can't spend the whole time just dealing with threats because we have to acquire resources to survive and also reproduce. So, we have to go out and find food, shelter and (as a social animal) friends and also partners to mate with – we can call these 'seeking emotions' or 'drive emotions' because they need to energise us to go out in the world and do and achieve things.

The third life task is that we can't spend all our time fighting or running away from threats or trying to achieve things. All living things have to find times to rest and recuperate.

When we recognise these three basic life tasks and challenges, we can see that we have three types of emotion that will help or sometimes hinder us. We have emotions that will help us to deal with detecting and responding to threats such as anger, anxiety or disgust. We have emotions that help us to seek out and achieve things such as interest, curiosity, excitement and the pleasure of consuming – these are mostly activating emotions. Thirdly, we have emotions and body states that help us to slow down, to settle and to be at rest.

Starting with the threat system (as that is usually the system that causes people the most difficulty), this system can be very fast acting and is all about protecting us. It will make us want to run away if something scares us, giving rise to the feeling of anxiety. It will make us want to attack or defend if we, or somebody we care about, are under threat (we feel this as anger), and it will make us want to get rid of anything that may poison us or give us a disease (disgust). One of the problems for humans is our ability to think and anticipate. So, for example, a zebra may get frightened and run away from a lion but it probably doesn't spend the rest of the day and evening ruminating about the problem of lions and what will happen if there's one about that it doesn't notice. The way we think about things and ruminate on things is a big stimulus for the threat system. In other words, our own thoughts, memories, worries and anticipations can all stimulate the threat system and keep us in loops of distress.

For the most part, threat emotions are designed to stop us doing things or to remove threat quickly. Because they're about stopping behaviours that could be harmful, the emotions are unpleasant and designed to try and remove the situation that's causing them. However, it's also the case that we can deliberately take on threats because we want to develop our skills and learn how to deal with our anxieties. For example, the first time you got into a car to learn to drive you were probably quite anxious, but you stayed with that anxiety because you wanted to achieve your goal. So, although threat emotions can be unpleasant, we can also learn how to tolerate them, work with them and develop our skills and abilities. Compassion is important because it helps to give us the courage to do this. It helps us develop our sense of self so that if we're struggling, we don't overly criticise ourselves, run ourselves down or constantly anticipate the worst. Rather, we focus on recognising the threat, recognising the emotions, and then working out what's going to be most helpful to deal with the situation and the emotion.

So, it's important to work out when our threats are helpful to us but also if we're ruminating or just avoiding things, as then threat emotions can become unhelpful. Similarly, if things make us angry and we are frightened of our anger and become very submissive, we might not be able to achieve the goals we want to. On the other hand, if we just become aggressive, this can be harmful to ourselves and others, so again it's learning how to work with and manage our threat emotions. For example, if we learn how to be helpfully assertive, how to promote our own values, how to make requests of people and how to stand up against the harmful behaviour of others, this can be more helpful than harmful.

The drive and the soothing/safeness system are both 'positive' emotion systems as they give us enjoyable feelings to encourage us to do more of these things.

The drive system gives us the energy and the motivation to go out and get what we need, such as food, a place to live, a partner, to achieve and to consume. It gives us a feeling of energy, excitement, anticipation and motivation. One of the core issues, however, is that the threat system can be triggered when we feel we can't achieve what we want to do. We feel we are struggling and trying but failing. Sometimes, we feel driven to achieve not because of the joy of doing so but because we want to avoid negative outcomes. For example, somebody may feel that if they don't achieve then other people will see them as a failure and lose interest in them in some way. Like all of our emotions then, there could be ways in which they can be helpful to us but also ways in which they can be unhelpful. When we practise compassion, we're learning how to use our drive emotions helpfully and how to pay attention to the pleasures of achievement rather than achievements always being about avoiding rejection or just needing to pay our rent or mortgage! In fact, the ability to generate positive emotion such as joyfulness, fun and playfulness can be very important for mothers because they can share these experiences with their children. Equally, when we're very tired, exhausted or doubting our abilities, generating that energy can be very difficult. When this happens, we can become self-critical and that can make it even more difficult. So, compassion helps us to be in tune with these processes so that we can begin to think about how we want to do things *that do* bring us pleasure; even small things like mindfully and purposefully cooking a meal we like, listening to music we like or contacting a friend. When some people are depressed, being able to do this can be hard because depression can knock out our abilities to feel positive emotion. As we will see throughout this book, these sorts of changes are not your fault, but the more we can understand them, the more we can effectively work on ways to help us with them.

There is a different type of positive emotion that's not based upon achieving or doing but simply upon feeling at peace with oneself – maybe just pottering about and enjoying the small things of life. Because this is not based on activation or an elevated positive emotion but instead on a quieter, more settled type of emotion, it's linked to what we call the rest and digest system. That means we're more likely to have these experiences if we are not over-stimulating our threat systems or drive systems or are caught up in feelings of inadequacy or needing to do or achieve more. Sometimes this is linked to what we call contentment or a form of settledness. This in turn is linked to a particular type of brain state.

What's interesting about this system is that it's also linked into how our social relationships work for us. Our relationships can stimulate it. For example, imagine a distressed baby and then the mother picks the baby up and the baby calms down. This is called soothing or settling, and the mother is literally settling the baby's threat and distress system through stimulating the rest and digest system – in a way enabling 'rest and calming'. The rest and digest, soothing, safeness system is activated when we have got what we need, when there is no threat, and when we feel safe. This safeness, for humans, is often social; for example, when we know that somebody thinks well of us.

No one system is better or worse than the others. We need to be able to draw upon all of them to function well in our lives. However, for many of us, our circumstances, backgrounds, illnesses, even our genes may mean that one particular pattern or circle is more dominant, or that one is particularly hard to access when we need it.

This workbook is all about learning ways to have a balance of all three systems. And to understand how to help our baby to have this balance too.

Let's look at these in more detail.

Module 6: The threat-protection system

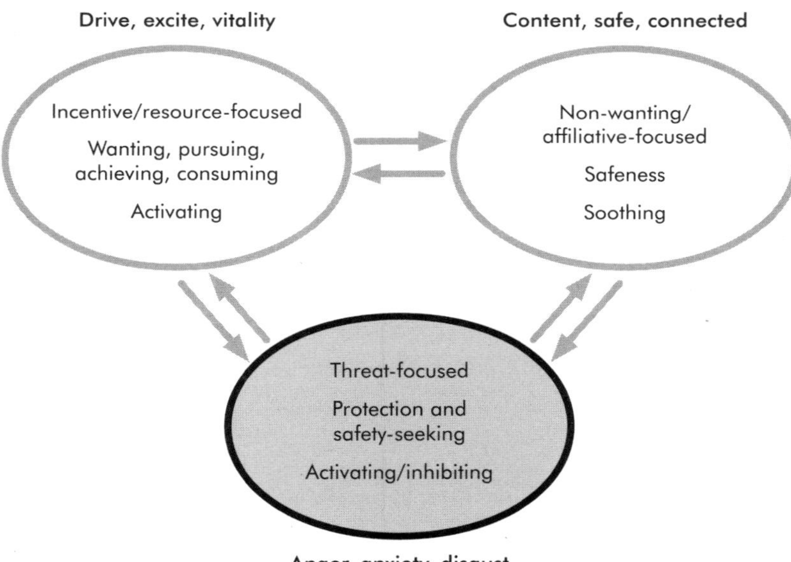

The system relating to threat protection (often coloured red in the diagram and sometimes referred to as the 'red system' or 'red circle') is the one that people are often most aware of, and it may be considered the system that is causing us problems and that needs controlling in some way. So, people may say that they want to learn to be able to feel less anxious or less angry for example. It is purposefully designed to produce unpleasant feelings and emotions in us so that we avoid threatening situations if at all possible, and so that we remember them vividly to avoid them in the future. This is because the threat system is concerned with keeping us safe.

It is designed to be activated at the slightest hint of danger. It even runs a 'better safe than sorry' policy so will alert us by raising our heart rate, speeding up our breathing and making us feel anxious or angry even when there is no threat, but where the brain perceives there might be. You might, for example, jump and freeze for a moment at a stick lying on the ground that your brain thought could be a snake. For our ancestors, those who didn't have this 'assume the worst/better safe than sorry' strategy within them were more likely to have been bitten by the snake (if it turned out to be one), so their more relaxed strategy wouldn't have been passed on. So it is not our fault that we assume the worst, jump to conclusions, find it hard to 'look on the bright side' and so on. These are powerful strategies passed on in our genes which helped our ancestors to survive and enabled us to be here, trying to work out how to help out our worried brain as best we can.

And what's more, the threat part of our old brain will cause us to react even before we become consciously aware of what just happened. It's not our fault and we can't do anything about the reaction apart from try to calm our brain and body down once we realise.

When was a time when your old brain reacted in this fast 'better safe than sorry' way before your new brain realised what was going on? (e.g. made you jump when your partner came quietly into the room, or went straight to anger when your baby accidentally hit you in the face with a toy)

____

____

____

____

____

The threat system is sometimes called the 'fight/flight' system because it is involved with the strategies of anger when we need to protect ourselves or something precious to us for example, and anxiety where the strategy is to avoid, move away, run away. However, there are not just these 'activating' strategies. We might also freeze in fear, or collapse in terror and become unable to speak, run away or fight. These are fast, automatic responses which happen before we can have control over them. They are not our fault.

We are going to look at the three threat responses of anxiety, anger and disgust in a bit more detail.

Anxiety

When was a time recently when you felt anxiety?

____

____

____

How did you know it was anxiety? What did you feel in your body?

____

____

____

What did your body really want to do if it could? What was the urge in your body?

____

____

____

How does your baby let you know when they are a little worried or fearful?

____

____

____

What seems to be the urge in your baby's body when they feel this way?

____

____

____

We can often tell by the urge in our body what the function of an emotion is. With anxiety, the urge is often to run away or avoid. It is usually a horrible feeling of a churning stomach, fast heart rate and fast breathing. You might also notice in your baby that they get upset and want close physical contact and reassurance. You might notice that you too would like contact with somebody and reassurance. If we re-look at the threat system circle in Figure 1 (Three circles), it says 'protection and safety seeking' – so not only does it alert us to danger, but the threat system also creates the urge within us to seek protection and safety.

There is a thought that we may have evolved to become more anxious when we are pregnant and have had a baby so that we become even more alert than usual to danger, particularly danger that may threaten our baby, but also that may threaten us now that we are the mother to the baby. However, some people report feeling calmer during pregnancy and once they have given birth, particularly if they are breastfeeding as this can have a calming effect because of the release of the hormone prolactin (unless breastfeeding is a difficult process, then of course it can create anxiety and frustration amongst other emotions. If this is the case don't struggle alone – your health visitor can put you in touch with breastfeeding advisors. There are also independent organisations that you can contact yourself such as La Leche League).

Have you noticed any changes in your general level of anxiety since becoming pregnant and having a baby?

____

____

____

If so, in what way?

____

____

____

If you are struggling with feeling very anxious, do let your midwife or health visitor know. There are services that can help you.

Anxiety that carries on for a while and is causing you problems can have many causes including hormone changes, feeling overwhelmed, exhaustion, lack of support, depression and post-traumatic stress disorder (PTSD) perhaps from a difficult birth. Whatever it may be, there are services set up to help you. You don't have to suffer with this. Especially when you are trying to look after a baby too.

Anger

When was a time recently that you felt irritation, frustration or anger?

____

____

____

How did you know this was the feeling? i.e. what was happening in your body?

____

____

____

If this feeling were to grow and grow, what would be the urge in your body? What would your body do if you let it?

____

____

____

When was a time recently when your baby appeared to be frustrated, irritable or angry?

____

____

____

How did you know this is what they were feeling?

____

____

____

If that feeling were to grow and grow in your baby, what do you imagine the urge might be in their body? What might they do if they could?

____

____

____

You might notice your heart and your breathing rate increase. Perhaps you notice tension in your body, perhaps clenching your jaw, or your fists. Your urge might be to shout, push or throw things. You might have a feeling of energy and strength. Again, the urge can give us an insight into the function of anger. So here we want to stop something happening to us, or to get something when we are being prevented from having it, for example. In our baby it might be about wanting something that they just can't get, for example a toy they can't reach. Or stopping something that they are not enjoying, such as being given one more spoonful of food when they are full.

Like all emotions, it is an important one in alerting us to problems and threats. It can sometimes be a hard emotion to experience, particularly in the perinatal period as we may worry that people won't want to be with us if we get angry with them. Or we might be scared of the impact on ourselves and our baby if they got angry with us in return. This could be a reality now. This of course would also have been a real source of vulnerability to us and our baby in our distant past when humans relied on the help of others to stay safe from predators and to acquire enough food for mother and baby. We still carry these ancient fears within us in terms of evolved fears and strategies that have kept us alive compared to people who didn't have these strategies. So, these strategies can still drive us now, even if logically we don't feel unsafe. It might mean that we try to suppress our anger or turn it in on ourselves using self-criticism, for example.

Have you noticed any changes in your general levels of anger, irritability or frustration since becoming pregnant or having a baby?

____

If so, in what way?

____

____

____

If you feel your anger levels are causing you difficulties then do see your midwife, health visitor or GP. There could be many reasons for this, including feeling overwhelmed by having a baby, feeling scared, lack of sleep, exhaustion, or the rapid hormonal changes involved in pregnancy, birth, breastfeeding and stopping breastfeeding. It can also be a symptom of depression or post-traumatic stress disorder (PTSD), for example. Whatever the cause, there are services that are set up to help you.

Disgust

If you look all the way back at Figure 1 (Three Circles), you see that under the threat circle, there aren't just the classic 'fight/flight' emotions of anger and anxiety. It also says 'disgust'. This threat emotion is often missed but is very important and can particularly come into play in the perinatal period.

Think about the last time you felt disgust. What happened to make you feel this way?

____

____

____

Where did you feel it in your body?

____

____

____

If the feeling were to grow and grow, what would be the urge? What would your body want to do if you really let it?

____

____

____

When did your baby last seem to experience disgust?

____

____

____

What had happened to make them feel this way?

____

____

____

What did they do?

____

____

____

Our urge once again can guide us to the function of disgust, and as ever, our baby can reveal it more clearly than we might see it as adults, as they don't yet have the self-consciousness to try to hide it. They can be great teachers to us adults who may have had a lifetime of trying to hide how we feel or of 'being polite'. In our baby, disgust may be connected to a food that they don't like. The function of disgust is to make sure we eject poisonous or gone-off food or to avoid things (or even people) that could introduce harmful viruses or bacteria to us. Babies develop other disgust responses socially, so they are not worried about touching their poo or picking their nose and eating it in public until they learn what is and isn't OK in their particular culture.

For some, we may feel that our body becomes disgusting to us during pregnancy, or that the feel of the baby moving inside us feels disgusting. We may experience pregnancy-related sickness as disgusting. For some, the birthing process makes us feel disgust and indeed can be the basis behind wishes to have a caesarean delivery.

And once the baby is born, having leaky breasts, lochia (the vaginal discharge after birth), constipation and so on can disgust some. Some find the thought of breastfeeding disgusting, and this can be behind the decision not to breastfeed.

Being hypersensitive to sensations, for example for some autistic people, can make pregnancy, birth, breastfeeding and the close physical contact and sensory demands of a baby difficult. The disgust response may be particularly heightened. (There are some online forums and support groups for autistic parents which can offer ways of managing these sensations. There is also more training available for health professionals to help understand these difficulties and to support solutions.)

Because we may have been taught to hide our disgust and 'be nice, be polite', it may be hard to identify that disgust is how we feel. And if we do feel disgust, we may not feel it is acceptable to say so. But if we can identify truly what is driving us, then we can much more accurately respond to it and try to help ourselves, or others, with it.

The experience of disgust is often given away by a curl of the lip and wrinkle of the nose that is associated with disgusting things, even if we, and others, may then label it as something else. So, we can pay attention to the body as it can reveal how we, and others, are really feeling, so that more appropriate action can be taken.

As our brains develop, we acquire the capacity to feel this disgust towards people (due to how they behave), and even towards ourselves. This can take the form of contempt; a kind of 'looking down on' and wanting to turn away from. It makes us want to stay away from a person and even to push them out of our group. Going back to the origins of us as humans, living in small groups navigating the threats of the African savannah, if we had a person who behaved in a way that really put our group at risk, or who behaved in a way that went against societal values that kept our group cohesive and safe, then we may experience them like a contaminant. The urge might be to eject them from the group, just like we eject harmful food. So, we can experience people as 'disgusting' too, feeling the same sensations of disgust, and the same urges to get rid of them.

But this of course has the flip side that we still carry with us; the in-built fear that *we* could be the one that the group wants to eject. We can therefore become disgusted with ourselves, contemptuous and self-critical, in an unconscious effort to correct ourselves before we become the type of person our group might want to cast out. Because of course if we were, for most of our human evolution, our survival chances on our own would be very low. And particularly so when we are pregnant or have a young baby. So, this is another reason why disgust, and also its link to self-criticism and self-contempt, can become even more heightened in the perinatal period. We will return to our self-critic later, as it doesn't usually work as we might hope or imagine it does. It can create deep misery in our lives. But there are some helpful ways of addressing our self-critic which we will look at in detail.

Do you ever feel disgust or contempt towards yourself?

This may be about a behaviour, thoughts or images you have. It may be towards particular emotions or urges.

____

____

____

What might your fear be if you didn't respond to it with disgust and just let it run?

____

____

____

One very common fear is that we would become a person that others wouldn't like. And the fear behind that is usually that then we would be alone, and of course then we are back to that primal fear; that we wouldn't survive. And neither would our baby. So we may notice that we have become even more critical of ourselves or others around this perinatal time. And this is not our fault at all.

Have you noticed this feeling of disgust or contempt towards any aspect of your baby, such as when they behave in a certain way, or exhibit a particular emotion? (Listen out for the words you might be saying in your head that might signal disgust – 'he is so clingy', 'stop crying like that; it's just pathetic' accompanied by that sneering, lip curled up, nose turned up facial expression.)

____

____

____

What might your fear be if they continued with this?

____

____

____

Sometimes we can be disgusted with our baby at things that disgust us about ourselves, or perhaps from early experiences of others who were treated with disgust or disgusted us in our family. We may fear that our baby might turn into a person whom people might reject, or who may 'contaminate' us and mean that we get rejected by association. It is an understandable fear. But, because disgust and contempt can be hard to notice, we may be trying to get rid of normal aspects of our baby that they really need in their life. For example, we may unconsciously regard clinginess in our baby with disgust and contempt, and try to stop them from being clingy, when in fact clinging on to their 'secure base' when they are scared is an important evolved survival strategy for babies and part of a secure attachment. We may also inadvertently give them a sense of shame about themselves for these normal things, perhaps like we were given too.

If we can identify our disgust reactions to our baby, and respond to ourselves with understanding and an urge to help, rather than shaming ourselves, then we can work out how to help ourselves with the very understandable fears that are actually the root cause of the disgust and contempt (more about how to do this later).

Your reflections and notes on this module about the threat system, and anger, anxiety and disgust.

What do you want to hold onto and remember? What would you like to take forward from here?

___

___

___

___

___

___

Module 7: The drive system

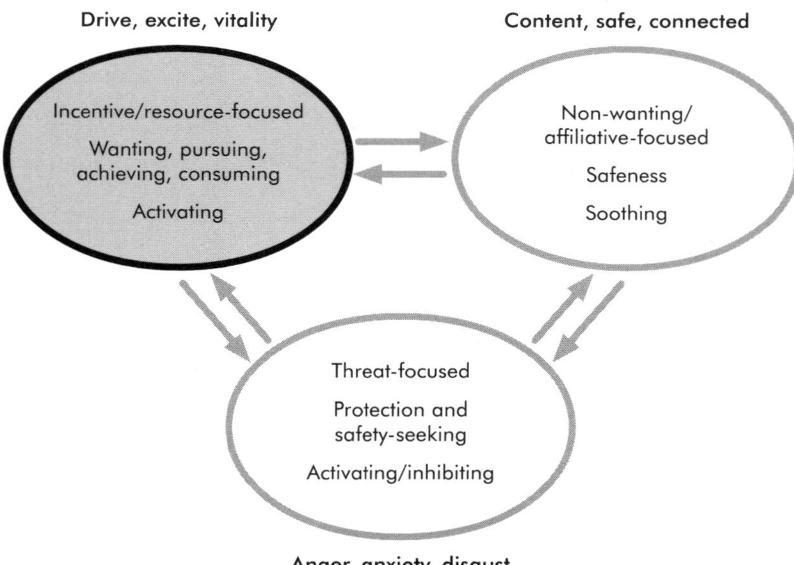

We are going to look at the first of the two 'positive' emotion systems now. This is the top left circle and is often referred to as the 'drive' or 'blue' system. If we think about a day in the life of a lizard, for example, it doesn't just defend itself from predators, run away to a safe place, or make sure it doesn't eat something poisonous (threat system), it also needs to go out and find food, a better place to live, and eventually a mate. It therefore needs a system that sets it off after its goal and gives it energy to do this, as well as the ability to have a narrowed focus on its goal so it remembers what it has set out to do.

We too of course have this system. We have this part of us that gets us moving to go and get what is needed, to achieve and to acquire. The emotions that help us with this are feelings of anticipation and excitement. It is a positive reward system to make sure we keep moving towards our goal. It is a very focused system, like the threat system, as it keeps us on track with the goal in our mind.

What were some of the things that you did today, from the moment of opening your eyes this morning?

____

____

____

What drove you to do them?

____

____

____

How did you feel when you achieved each one?

____

____

____

What makes it easier to do these things?

____

____

____

What makes it harder?

____

____

____

What have you noticed your baby wanting to do since they woke up this morning?

____

____

____

How do they react when they manage to get or achieve it?

____

____

____

How do they react if something gets in the way of their goal?

____

____

____

Our baby shows us the drive system at its simplest and most uncomplicated; be near someone who settles you, have food, be made comfortable, do interesting things, learn, make relationships. In your day, especially with a baby, the drive system is probably going at high speed. There may be moments of pleasure when something is achieved, but the main motivation may be to stay out of the threat system, for example to keep on top of things to avoid feeling overwhelmed and in chaos.

Imagine if you lived in a time or a place where you had people around you who shared the care of your baby with you. (This is how we lived for most of our human life. And what is more, they actively wanted to, because a new baby is a precious and much-needed addition to a tribe.)

What might your drive system look like now?

____

____

____

Perhaps there would be different things to do and achieve. Maybe it would feel a little calmer. Perhaps there might be more time to do the things that bring you joy, rather than focusing solely on what might reduce your threat system, as we generally tend to do. Perhaps there might be more threat, such as getting enough food, or trying to stay alive through a harsh winter.

But when we do share in the care of our baby, as we are wired to do, then we can feel freed up to spend time having more playful and joyful interactions with our baby, and to be able to focus on longer-term goals such as building our baby's sense of confidence, skills and so on, to be able to go out into the world when they grow up.

We can also have some time to feed what keeps us functioning well too.

This motivation system is a very complicated neurobiological set-up. There is a whole area of science investigating just what happens, even prior to the moment we have the conscious thought 'I need to get up and go and do this', let alone what gives us the 'oomph' to actually set things in motion.

It is not surprising then that it can be knocked off course. Depression is something that particularly takes down the drive system. Even feeling a bit low or fed up can make it feel hard to get up and do anything. Depression takes this even further and can make the world feel 'grey' rather than in colour. Things can feel 'pointless'. *We* can even feel pointless. And this is just because this particular physiological system has been disrupted for one reason or another. But we can believe the thoughts that arise through the disruption of this system. We can believe them to such a degree because they seem like the truth, so much so that sometimes tragically people can believe it as fact that their family would be better off without them. It feels like it is true just because of the biology of our motivational system and how it responds to depression. When these thoughts come about it is regarded as 'a medical emergency' and help needs to be given as soon as possible, via the GP, calling the NHS helpline (111), going to Accident and Emergency or calling an ambulance (999) if you, or the person affected, feels unable to keep themselves safe. There are perinatal Mother and Baby units available all around the country, set up for mothers experiencing severe mental illness in pregnancy or postnatally, and depression is treatable. You and your baby will be looked after until you are well.

When we have postnatal depression, it is incredibly difficult to have the energy or desire to look after oneself, let alone our baby. Even our ability to do the 'to and fro' interactions with our baby can feel difficult and 'clunky' when we feel depressed, as even these interactions require some input from the drive system. This is why it is so important to get help from your health visitor or GP, and why perinatal mental health services in the UK are having so many resources put into them; to prioritise the mental and physical health of mothers. It is also why sharing the care with others is so important, particularly whilst recovering from depression.

It is still possible to interact well with our baby, even when we have depression, but we may need help with this, and we need treatment for the depression. So please don't suffer quietly with depression, hoping it will go away. Seek help quickly, even if it is to talk over with your GP or health visitor whether you do have postnatal depression and whether you need some support with interacting with your baby. It can feel a great relief, and treatment can often be relatively quick but can have a potentially far-reaching impact for you and your baby.

Your reflections and notes on this module about the drive system.

What do you want to hold onto and remember? What would you like to take forward from here?

____

____

____

____

Module 8: The soothing and safeness system

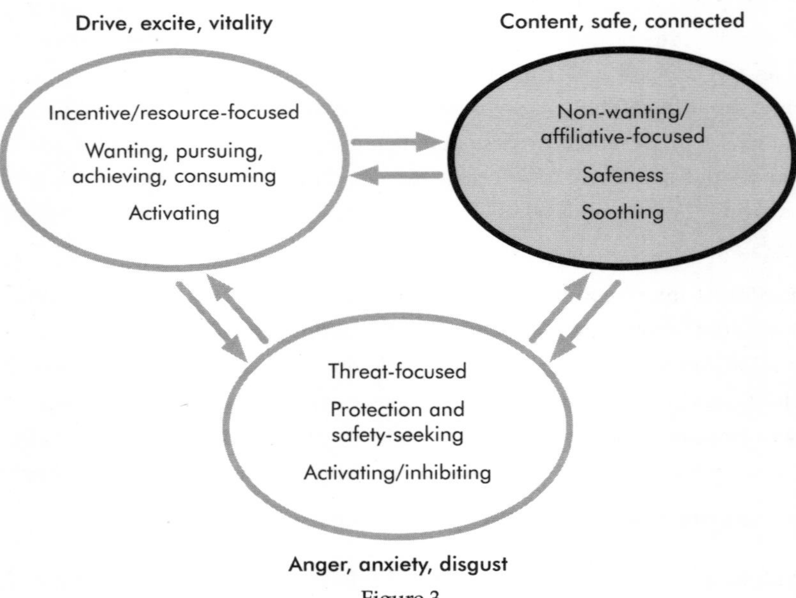

Figure 3

The soothing and safeness system (often coloured green in the diagram and sometimes called the 'green system' or 'green circle') is the system we are in when there are no threats to be dealing with (so the threat system isn't activated) and there is nothing that we need right now (so the drive system isn't activated), giving us a feeling of calm and contentment, enabling us to rest, digest and recuperate. It might seem like the absence of drive and threat will automatically move us into our soothing/safeness system (it certainly helps). But we also need to have a sense of safeness. For humans, this usually comes from social connection;

from knowing that there are people who care about us and will help us if we need it. When we have this, we feel calm, contented, settled and steady. It is this system which supports our care-giving and care-receiving motivations and the new brain extension of this – compassion.

Bring to mind a time when someone was kind to you. It might just be a fleeting moment such as an understanding smile when your baby is crying in the supermarket, the midwife taking hold of your hand when you were struggling during delivery of your baby, a thoughtful text message from someone.

How do you feel in your body as you remember this?

____

____

____

We can see that even just recalling a memory of kindness to us is enough to stimulate our soothing / safeness system; our breathing and heart rate slow down, we may feel calmer and steadier, just from a memory.

What switches on your baby's soothing/safeness system?

____

____

____

How do you know that they are in their soothing/safeness system? What do you notice in them?

____

____

____

You might notice that when your baby is feeling soothed and safe, they look at you, at other faces, and at their surroundings. This is because when we feel soothed and safe our mind and body work in very different ways to when we are in threat or drive (it applies to us too, not just our baby). Rather than having a narrow focus on the threat or the object of our drive system, we can now have a wide focus of attention. We actually look at things differently. And we can also take in this new learning and integrate it into what we already know. Even the part of our brain involved is different. When we feel safe, we are more able to use our pre-frontal cortex, a part of our evolutionarily 'new brain' housed approximately behind our eyebrows. This part of the brain is involved in helping us to learn, be creative and understand the minds of others, pulling together information into a clear picture (integration), our sense of who we are (sense of self) and even our values – the person that we want to be. So, although experiencing safeness is something that our 'old brain' responds to, it opens up a gateway into the pre-frontal cortex of our 'new brain' and all the incredible mental abilities that we then have access to.

Imagine you are trying to get out of the house with your baby. You are late for your appointment, and your baby is refusing to have their hat on. It's a cold day.

What happens if you start getting stressed?

____

____

____

What happens if you can breathe deeply, slow down a bit and calm down?

____

____

____

You might notice that when we are in threat, we tend to get stuck using one strategy because our threat brain becomes narrowly focused. We might find ourselves just wanting to keep putting the hat on and getting crosser, for example.

When we can calm down and slow down, it is as if the pre-frontal part of our 'new brain' becomes 'unlocked'. Now it is easier to think of different strategies ('I'll put the rain cover on so at least it's a bit warmer in the buggy' or 'If I give her this toy, she won't notice that I've put her hat on', or 'I wonder if perhaps this hat has got a bit small and uncomfortable for him? Perhaps it's time for a new one').

It is also easier to put it into perspective – 'Actually she is pretty snug in her buggy, and we won't be out very long so it's probably not such a big deal.'

As we will see, the soothing/safeness system really does do some incredible things.

When we feel soothed and safe, our brain works differently:

We move from a narrow focus of attention in threat to a wide focus of attention.

We are better able to learn new things.

We can find creative solutions,

and see things from other people's points of view more easily –

including our baby.

The power of the soothing and safeness system

The safeness and soothing system can sometimes be viewed mistakenly as the relaxation system, or the 'having-some-me-time' system. These things are of course important and there are elements of resting and settling and also taking care of oneself. But if this is solely how we see this system then we might disregard its importance, particularly if, for example, there is no time to relax or have time for ourselves now we have a baby, or if we feel we don't deserve time for ourselves, or if we fear that if we did take it then we'd lose momentum and might never get up and look after the baby again.

We are going to see just how profoundly important this system is – not just for our own functioning, but also for being able to parent at our best.

Imagine there is a baby happily playing on the floor at a clinic with his parent next to him. Suddenly a fire alarm goes off.

What does the baby do?

He might startle, start to cry, turn to his parent and put his arms up to be picked up.

Which of the three circles is he now in? (Which emotional system?)

The threat system.

How do you think his parent will react to him?

They might pick him up, hold him close, reassure him.

What happens now to the baby?

The baby is likely to calm down, stop crying, perhaps start to look around, point, babble or talk if they are at these developmental stages.

So, which of the three circles is the baby now in?

___

___

___

The baby is probably now in their soothing/safeness system.

What we see here is that even if the fire alarm was still going off, the parent can settle the baby. They have detected the signals of their baby's distress and been motivated to alleviate the distress (care-giving/compassion motivational system). They pick up and soothe the baby, which has then switched on the baby's own soothing/safeness system.

The soothing/safeness system turns down and settles the threat system.

This is key; even when a threat remains, as social animals, we have evolved for our threat systems to be regulated by the detection of safeness, which includes the presence of another person whom we perceive as safe and helpful.

We have evolved for the stresses of life to be regulated through social contact.

And as we see with the baby in this example, it doesn't just turn down our threat system so that we are calmer, but it also helps us to use a different part of our brain. For the baby, when he was in his threat system he was totally focused on the threat and on finding safeness. But once he was safe, the pre-frontal part of his brain was freed up and he could look around, start to integrate any new information into his pre-existing knowledge and even be able to begin playing again and being creative.

Of course this doesn't just apply to our baby. We never grow out of the impact that feeling safe has on our brain and our body. And no matter how much we learn to settle and soothe ourselves, still the fastest and most powerful way of feeling settled and safe after feeling angry or scared is by compassion from other people.

This is why this book teaches how to both bring compassion to ourselves to self-soothe and settle, but also to look to others for help and support, and importantly, to be able to allow ourselves to accept and take in that help and support when it is offered (which for many can be much harder than it might sound).

Imagine that, in the above example, the fire alarm was turned off, but the baby wasn't picked up.

How would the baby be?

____

____

____

____

The baby might stay upset, and even if he stopped crying, he might still be looking for the threat to return. He probably will not go back to playing, or if so, will remain wary. In other words, he is still in his threat system.

How long might the baby remain upset or wary if he is not picked up?

____

____

____

____

He might well stay upset or hypervigilant for a long time. We can compare this to just how quickly a baby or an adult calms down when they experience safeness from others or from themselves, as opposed to just having the threat removed but no signals of safeness received.

This really highlights just how crucial our soothing/safeness system is. When we experience threat, we of course imagine that we need to focus on getting rid of the threat (and we do). But what can get missed, especially if we haven't had this ourselves, is that our main way of calming back down and being able to carry on with our lives is by having our soothing/safeness system switched on – either by others, or by us. Without the soothing/safeness system, we stay on red alert, even when there is no threat. This also applies to our baby. Which is why the presence of someone who represents safeness – their 'secure base and safe haven' – is so vital to them, helping to keep them not just psychologically well, but physically well too. (We will look a bit more at this in the section on 'uncertainty'.)

Without the soothing/safeness system we stay on red alert.

Even when there is no threat.

The difference between 'safety' and 'safeness'

We often use the words 'safety' and 'safeness' to mean the same thing. In fact, there is an important distinction.

Safety is to do with detecting whether there is a threat and is part of the threat system. Even if we don't detect a threat, we can still be on alert. For example, even at night we may struggle to sleep because part of our brain is 'listening' for our baby waking up.

Safeness, on the other hand, is when we are detecting signals that we are safe, and all is well. For humans, these signals are often social, for example a kind smile from somebody in the supermarket when our baby is crying. Safeness is connected to the soothing/safeness system rather than the threat system. We feel this as a kind of breathing out and ease in our body. We see this for our baby too – that even if there is no threat, it is not until they are in our arms or know that we are near that we see their body relax. Compassionate mind work is all about creating safeness, for example by helping us to create relationships that we feel settled and secure in, but also by creating our own internal compassionate mind that helps us to feel settled and safe inside.

My examples of safety:

____

____

____

e.g. checking that all the doors are locked at night. Asking my health visitor for reassurance about my baby. Keep checking on my baby in the night. My self-critic starts up to make sure I don't get too loud and annoy people when I go to the parent and baby group. Making sure the neighbours aren't outside when I go out.

How do I know this is safety rather than safeness for me?

____

____

____

e.g. I feel like I'm 'on edge'. My heart is beating quite fast still. I can't quite switch my mind off. I feel a bit like I've forgotten something that I needed to do. I still feel like I could do with some reassurance. I feel like I'm holding my breath a bit.

My examples of safeness:

____

____

____

e.g. when my partner comes home. When I have just done the 'big shop', and I have everything I need in the house. When I am seated with my dog on the sofa. When Mum takes the baby out for a walk, and I know he is in good hands. Knowing there are people I can phone if I need to, but at the moment it's just nice to sit on my own watching TV whilst the baby is sleeping. Having a really nice message from a friend that I was worried I had upset.

How do I know it is safeness rather than safety for me?

___

___

___

e.g. I feel like I've just breathed out properly. My body feels looser and more at ease. My mind can 'switch off' and I can watch this programme on TV or read my book properly now. I can think of new ideas and come up with solutions to things. I feel calm. I feel joyful. I am looking forward to seeing particular people.

What is the difference between safety and safeness for my baby?

Safety:

___

___

___

e.g. their body stiffens up. They stop playing and just watch in an intense rather than curious way. They look for me or my partner. They look serious.

Safeness:

___

___

___

e.g. they smile. They make happy noises. Their body relaxes. They do a poo. They snuggle up and feel heavy. They get engrossed in playing. They look around in interest. They 'chat' away to me and the cat and have a 'conversation' with us.

What is the difference between safety and safeness for my partner?

Safety:

Busying around, doing jobs in a slightly stressed manner, serious face, not very relaxed. Keep checking their emails. Not very chatty to me and the baby.

Safeness:

Smiley, cuddly, sitting with ease with me and the dog on the sofa, looking forward to seeing his friends. Chatting to me and the baby. Talking about things we are looking forward to doing as a family in the future.

Your reflections and notes on this module about the soothing and safeness system, the power of this system and the difference between safety and safeness.

What do you want to hold onto and remember? What would you like to take forward from here?

Module 9: The relative sizes of our three circles

So now we have looked at the three circles or systems, which is the circle that your baby currently spends the largest part of their day in?

____

Which circle do they spend the least amount of their day in?

____

Draw the relative sizes of their three circles in the box below (how big would the biggest circle be compared to their smallest?):

Relative sizes of your baby's three circles in a typical day at the moment:

What do you imagine this is like for your baby? How do the relative sizes of their systems play out in their lives?

____

____

____

How do you help your baby to move between their three circles?

____

____

____

How has the relative sizes of your baby's three circles changed since they were born?

____

____

____

Babies often sleep a lot in the early weeks, as they are processing such a lot of new information. They are likely to want to be secure in someone's arms or snug in a familiar place to sleep. So, they are largely in their soothing/safeness system. Unfortunately, some babies cry a lot, for example if they suffer from colic, so they (and we) may spend a lot of time in threat. (Do seek help from your health visitor if this is the case. There is also the organisation Cry-sis that can be very helpful, and there may be other local and national organisations too if you are able to search the internet. Local groups of parents can also be a good source of help and support, such as your local Parent and Toddler group.)

As our baby gets older, they are likely to spend more time in drive, exploring the world and the people around them. But to do this they need to feel safe too. So here the drive and the soothing/safeness system go hand-in-hand. They can sometimes get a bit overwhelmed by too much stimulation and so may move into threat, demonstrating this by becoming crotchety and disgruntled, needing you to perhaps pick them up, settle and soothe them. As you stimulate their soothing/safeness system, this then calms their threat system back down.

Sometimes they may get bored when the drive system isn't stimulated enough, so they begin dropping into the threat system, again getting crotchety and cross. Here, rather than needing soothing (unless they have got too upset), they just need more stimulation – a different toy, singing some songs with you, being taken to look at something out of the window, having a look at a book with you, 'helping' you put the washing in the washing machine, and so on.

Phew. So, this is what we are doing all day as a parent. Such a skill, often without realising it – regulating our baby, but also learning how to regulate *our* baby, who may be different to our own character, or to other people we are familiar with. And on top of that trying to keep up with learning how they now need to be regulated as they grow older. Often, we just manage to catch up with their changes when they've moved on again. Pretty amazing really, what we're doing.

Of course we won't be doing this perfectly, as this is impossible, and if we were somehow able to, our baby wouldn't be learning how to tolerate the 'gaps' where they experience a little bit of discomfort while we work out how to help them. Indeed the whole experience of synchrony (which we will look at later) is about our efforts to move back into matched behaviour and then the moving out again – it is constant ebb and flow, and it is really our *intention and efforts* to be holding the baby in mind, and understand what they are trying to tell us, and respond as best we can, that is the most important thing.

We see particularly in our baby that they really enjoy interacting face to face with us for a short while, but then break our gaze and look away. This is because babies become easily over-stimulated and need time to regulate again and to process all that interaction, laying it down as new memories. When they are ready, they will bring their gaze back again. This can be a bit disconcerting if we don't realise this – we can mistakenly think that we are boring to them or that they don't like us, and then we either work harder to engage them, or can mentally or physically withdraw – both of which are difficult for the baby and for us. So, we just need to let our baby pause, look away and then come back – finding ease and enjoyment in the looseness of this. Breathe in, breathe out slowly, become more loose, at ease, and just watch and follow your baby – they will let us know what they need.

So just let your baby pause, look away and then come back – finding ease and enjoyment in the looseness of this – for both your baby and you.

Breathe in, breathe out slowly, become more loose, at ease, and just watch and follow your baby – they will let you know what they need.

Although it is important not to deliberately leave a baby in discomfort, particularly when they are very young, the inevitable 'gaps' of life when you cannot respond immediately when they are older enable them to learn that these minor levels of discomfort don't mean they are going to fall apart, or disintegrate or die. They learn that they can bear some discomfort, and that help will arrive shortly. They will also learn that even if their parent can't remove the threat (for example, if their head hurts after banging it as they try to stand up under a table), it somehow feels a whole lot better when they are held, and soothed and have someone who is motivated to 'try' and wants to make it better – they are learning the power of compassion and the soothing / safeness system.

When you respond to your baby's distress they learn that even if you can't stop the hurt (e.g. a bumped head), it feels a whole lot better just by having someone who is trying to help as best they can.

This is the power of compassion and the soothing/safeness system.

They are learning that there are people who care about them and want to help them, and that they are lovable and worthy of help. They are learning that they can be helped, and that they have reliable strategies within themselves to get that help (self-efficacy and self-agency). What a lot they learn from us picking them up when they bang their head.

And this learning gets laid down in their memories, their brain connections and their body. Even their genes. It is the basis of their own compassionate mind, which they will use for themselves as they grow older, and to help others, and importantly too – to be able to take in the help that others offer them.

This experience of safeness from us gets laid down in our baby's memories, their brain connections, their body. Even their genes.

It is the basis of their own compassionate mind.

Ways of increasing soothing for your baby (and you)

- Proximity (being nearby may be enough, touch, stroking, holding, tucking them in close to you)
- Rocking
- Feeding
- Explaining, even if they can't understand – babies from a young age respond to voice tone and facial expression just as we do
- Naming emotions as they get older – this calms the amygdala in all of us (the amygdala is part of the threat system)
- Feeling your breath slowing down as you hold them against your chest – regulating their breath
- Deep-voiced slow singing that vibrates the chest
- Singing
- Toning (a single, deep, long, slow 'Ou' or 'Om' sound on your out breath that vibrates your chest and can be calming for you and your baby)
- Gentle dancing
- Being silly and having fun
- A quiet and darker environment
- Giving them their favourite toy to hold
- Stroking their cat or dog
- Going outside
- A ride in the pushchair or car
- A bath
- White noise, e.g. the sound of a fan whirring or washing machine going
- Watching a favourite TV programme with you
- Having a story read to them
- Snuggling with a different person if you are feeling stressed
- Being taken to a different room with you for a change of scenery

What helps your baby to be soothed?

____

____

____

When do you find it easiest to soothe your baby?

____

____

____

When do you find it hardest to soothe your baby?

____

____

____

We often find it hardest to soothe and settle our baby when we feel tired, irritable, pre-occupied, overwhelmed. In other words, it is very difficult to move our baby out of their threat system and into their soothing system when we are in our own threat system. We tend to find it a whole lot easier to soothe our baby if we feel rested, calm and steady ourselves. In other words, the system we are in is absolutely key when we are trying to change the system that our baby is in. So, we need to feel safe, soothed and settled in order to settle and soothe our baby.

We need to feel safe, soothed and settled in order to settle and soothe our baby.

Oxygen mask principle

There might be many reasons why it is sometimes harder and sometimes easier to soothe our baby. One big difference though is how exhausted, depleted, worried, hungry or in a hurry we feel. In other words, the system or circle that we are in has a profound impact on our ability to be with and soothe our baby when they are upset. If we are in our threat system, for whatever reason, then we are in a different part of the brain to the one needed for soothing and connection. No wonder we then find soothing others hard.

If we look back at the three circles diagram, it says 'safety seeking' in the threat circle. So, when we are in threat, our motivational system is to find safety, which might be someone who can help and support *us*. This is where the oxygen mask principle comes in. When you travel on a plane, in the safety announcement they say that you must put the oxygen mask on yourself before you put one on your child.

Why do you think this is?

____

____

____

This is because if we don't have enough oxygen, then we simply cannot help our child. This is the same when we are in threat – we need to put the oxygen mask of kindness and compassion on ourselves first.

When we do, then we feel settled and soothed. We have actually switched systems from threat to soothing. Now we can bring our soothing system, and the motivational systems that come from this of care-giving and compassion, rather than our threat system, to our distressed baby.

> *When we are in threat, we need to put the oxygen mask of kindness and compassion on ourselves first.*

We might say, 'but that takes too long', and that is the dilemma. But if we don't take even a moment, or one deep in and one long slow out breath, or some kind words to ourselves

– 'This is hard. You are doing so well' – then we will carry on trying to deal with our baby from threat, which rarely gets us a soothed baby or a soothed self.

Which circle is the one *you* spend a large part of your day in?

___

___

___

Which do you spend the least part of your day in?

___

___

___

Draw the relative sizes of your three circles in the box below:

Did your three circles look anything like this?

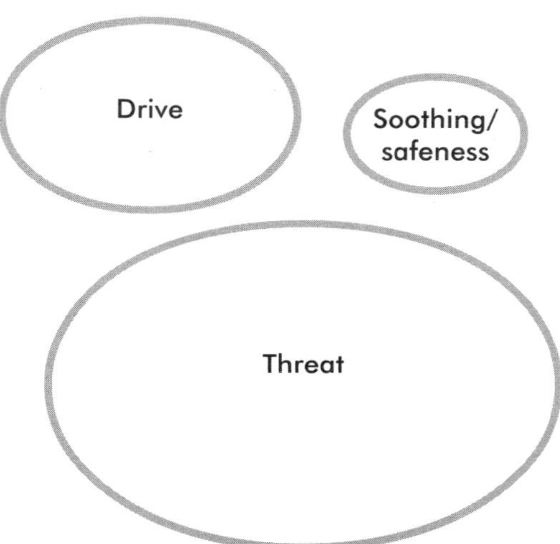

This is a typical picture that people draw when asked to do this exercise. The relative sizes of our three circles of course depend on many things and will be changing moment to moment, but we are just thinking about whether, on the whole, in our life over the last few days or weeks, we have one much more dominant emotional regulation system and one much smaller one. If we feel overwhelmed with things to do, then our threat and drive system may be equally large, and our soothing system quite small. If we feel a little low or depressed, our threat system may be large and both our drive and soothing systems small. Or perhaps we feel quite worried or frustrated about things; here our threat circle may be the biggest of the three. Maybe mostly we feel 'in balance' where sometimes we worry, but we can get things done, and we can also feel settled and soothed – where no circle is really dominant.

What would you put in your threat system? What is currently making you feel frustrated, angry or worried?

____

____

____

What would you put in your drive system? What motivates you? What are you moving towards or trying to achieve in your day/in your life at the moment? What excites you/makes you happy/brings you joy or satisfaction as you move towards achieving it?

____

____

____

What would you put in your soothing/safeness system? What makes you feel settled, calm, contented/gives you a feeling of breathing out, of being at ease?

____

____

____

Your partner's three circles

Draw below what you think are the relative sizes of your partner's three circles:

The relative sizes of your partner's three circles:

Write in the circles what you think would be

1. **Sources of threat for them**
2. **Sources of drive for them**
3. **Sources of soothing, safeness and contentment for them**

Looking back at what you have put in for your three circles, how do you and your partner's three circles interact?

____

____

____

What happens to the other person's three circles when each of you is in:

Threat?

____

____

____

Drive?

____

____

____

Soothing/safeness?

____

____

____

How do the three circles of both you and your partner interact with the three circles of your baby:

When your baby is in threat?

____

____

____

When your baby is in drive?

____

____

____

When your baby is in soothing/safeness?

____

____

____

We can see how our three systems are interacting with those of the people we share our lives with. How our systems interact is not our fault but the outcome of so many factors that we didn't choose, including our genes, the environment we were brought up in, even experiences that happened to our grandparents that get passed on to us in our genes. This is about stepping back and really noticing what is going on between the people in our lives, without judgement and with compassion. If we can hold what we observe in this honest and caring way, then we can see more clearly what it might be helpful to tweak and change. Hopefully, you and your partner will find many helpful things in this book that will aid with this process of change.

If your three circles feel 'out of balance'

It is very rare that anybody complains of feeling too at ease or too content so this section will assume that by 'out of balance' this refers to a disproportionately large threat system or, occasionally, drive system. When our threat system is large, we assume that we have too much anger or too much anxiety. We may seek out help for 'anger management' or 'anxiety management'. This may be helpful. However, if we remember the example of the baby at the clinic scared by the fire alarm, we saw here that the baby needed picking up and soothing and it was this stimulation of their soothing system that calmed and regulated their threat system. If the baby wasn't picked up, he would stay on red alert even when the threat had gone. This is the same for us as adults. We also need to be receiving signals of safeness to have our threat systems calmed and regulated. These are often social safeness signals such as reassurance from somebody we trust or remembering what a good friend or trusted family member might say to us in that situation.

And just like the baby, if *we* don't have access to these signals of safeness from outside of us, or inside of us, then we can stay in a state of anxiety or anger for a long time. We may feel uneasy or find it hard to calm down, even though logically we know the threat is no longer there.

What are new sources of soothing, safeness and contentment that you have discovered since having your baby? (Perhaps new friends, feeding your baby, enjoying the opportunity to go out for a walk with your baby during the day, feeling closer to a particular family member . . .)

____

____

____

What are sources of safeness, soothing and contentment that you feel like you may have lost or are finding it harder to get, now you have a baby? For example, friends at work that you don't see very much now, struggling to find time to go for a walk or a run on your own, finding it hard to read a book, or do some crafts . . .

____

____

____

It may seem unhelpful to think about what we might have lost, or struggle to get now, but sometimes we can feel out of sorts when we have our baby and assume that it is tiredness, or that we are struggling with being a mother, or with our baby. In fact, rather than it being the *arrival* of a threat, it might be the *loss* of what regulates us and soothes us that is the issue. Once we know this, we can now redirect our attention from trying to reduce the threat (although this might be needed too) to increasing our sources of soothing and safeness. Even if we can't get them at the moment, we can work towards it, as well as looking out for new sources of soothing and safeness.

When we feel really out of sorts it can feel like we need an enormous amount in the soothing system to have any chance of calming our oversized threat system. However, just like when we are thirsty we might feel like we could drink a lake's worth of water, actually after just a glass or two the thirst vanishes. Or when we are so tired we feel we need to sleep for a week, but after just one or two good nights of sleep we feel transformed. This is the same with our threat system – it doesn't need that much input from the soothing system to calm back down. So, we may feel that we need a week's break from our baby to rejuvenate, but actually a night with our partner in front of the TV with the baby being looked after elsewhere can suddenly make us feel a whole lot better. Even a break of thirty minutes to ourselves can restore us more than we might think. So rather than think, 'Oh that will only give me five minutes, it's not worth it', take the five minutes. It really doesn't take long to switch systems from threat to soothing.

Let's go back to your drawing of the relative sizes of your three circles. If your soothing system has been drawn very small, how do you manage your threat system when you really only have your threat and your drive system to operate through? When you feel anxious or angry, what do you do to manage this?

___

___

___

When people only really have their drive system at their disposal to manage threat, then these are some of the things they do to manage states of anger or anxiety:

- Taking the baby out of the house all the time – not because this is enjoyable but because being in the house is more anxiety provoking

- Cleaning a lot – in a threat-driven way – and even when it is all clean, still feeling unsettled or on high alert that it is going to get messed up again
- Exercising beyond what feels healthy
- Eating for comfort
- Undereating for achievement or out of anger
- Trying so hard to be doing what a 'perfect' mother does that they feel exhausted and resentful
- Using alcohol/sweet foods/drugs/self-harm to bring a feeling of relief, happiness, dulling the difficult feelings
- Seeking relationships that give a 'hit' of contact with someone but are ultimately harmful
- Buying things that make them feel good in the moment, but wish they hadn't bought even a few hours later

What is so sad about this list is that when we think about what people hope to feel if they do these things, it is usually to feel relief, at ease, safe, settled, content. So intuitively people are trying to get to the soothing system. However, because this system is so tiny, and there may not be the memories or the experience of knowing how to switch on and grow this system, the only motivational systems available are to avoid or shut down threat, or to try to do more/achieve more/eat more/buy more. As the soothing system has not been activated and the threat system is still in control, the outcome is still one of feeling anxious or angry, now perhaps joined by a helping of shame too.

Your reflections and notes on this section about the relative sizes of our 'three circles' for us, our baby and our partner, and what happens when they are out of balance.

What do you want to hold onto and take forward?

____

____

____

____

____

Like with the baby in the clinic with the fire alarm; to calm the threat system we need to activate the soothing system. So how do we do this when we are in threat? We need to go through a series of steps. There are five key steps that we are going to look at in detail here. Although we are going to spend a bit of time on each one so that we are clear about the rationale behind it, once we get the hang of it, it will only take a few minutes to go through all five. Each one is like a stepping stone, taking us across from the threat system to the soothing system.

Module 10: The five stepping stones from threat to soothing and safeness: 1) Posture

A note on the sympathetic and parasympathetic nervous system and their importance in compassionate mind work

To really understand what we are trying to do with our compassionate mind, it helps to understand our biology. A key part of this is our autonomic nervous system (ANS), which controls many aspects of us including our heart rate, breathing and gut.

- The out breath is controlled by the parasympathetic nervous system (PNS). It is linked to slowing down our heart rate and puts the 'brakes' on the threat system.
- The threat system (and the drive system) is connected to the sympathetic part of the autonomic nervous system (ANS). This sympathetic nervous system (SNS) is connected to speeding up our breathing and our heart rate, and getting us ready for action such as 'flight, fight or excite'.
- The sympathetic nervous system is the one most 'in charge' when we are in threat or drive.
- In our compassionate mind work, we are trying to stimulate our parasympathetic nervous system in many different ways as this is what allows us to rest, digest, recuperate and feel soothed and safe. It is also the system that supports care-giving, care-receiving and compassion.

Stepping stone one: Posture

For this section we will be looking at just how important our body is in all of this. To do this it is more helpful to move our body than to just read about it. So, read through each section, do the exercise, then jot down what you notice.

First of all, stand up and hang your head down as if you feel really heavy, letting your arms hang heavily too. Notice . . .

. . . how this feels in your body.

____

____

____

. . . what you can see.

. . . the thoughts that are running through your mind.

. . . how you feel in yourself emotionally.

Anything else you notice?

Now, very slowly and mindfully stand upright. Now what do you feel in your body?

What can you see?

____

____

____

What thoughts are running through your mind?

____

____

____

How do you feel in yourself emotionally?

____

____

____

Anything else you notice?

____

____

____

There are of course individual differences in how people respond to these two body positions, but generally, when people are in the hanging down position, they report feeling heavy in mood, finding breathing restricted, that they can only see their feet and a bit of the ground, and that even their thoughts become a bit more negative. (As we will see later, some feel safer and more protected in the hanging down position.)

Submissive versus dominant body posture

When people then stand upright, they tend to report feeling lighter in mood, more energised, more confident, able to breathe more freely, the room seems lighter, thoughts are more positive, and they can now see lots of things including other people (if there are people there with us).

All this from just changing our body posture. When we hang down, this signals to our brain that we are in a submissive posture. We see this most clearly in other mammals, including dogs who will roll over on their back revealing their belly, with eyes and ears back. In humans, a submissive posture is usually head down, eyes averted, body more slumped and displaying a lack of energy. This submissive posture is a vital safety strategy that is still preserved within humans because it has been so successful in keeping us safe. Like with the dog, it is a fast signal to the dominant individual that we have registered that we are weaker or less dominant, so don't attack us. The dominant individual is then able to save energy and possible injury so is more likely to leave without attacking. It literally saves lives, so gets passed on in our genes. When we hang down, we send signals up to our brain that makes it think we are under attack, so our threat system gets switched on and we feel anxious. It even reduces our energy and drive system so that we can't attack.

On the other hand, when we stand upright, we are adopting a more confident posture (not dominant, though) and our brain registers that all must be well and switches on the soothing/safeness system, which calms the threat system. We feel more energetic, positive, calm and steady. All by changing our posture.

When we stand upright in an open, confident posture (even if we don't feel confident but just change our body posture), this switches on our soothing/safeness system and calms the threat system.

All by changing our posture.

This overlaps with the fascinating research on testosterone. Testosterone levels were measured, then people were asked to either stand or sit with arms dangling, legs crossed and head down. Or to stand or sit upright with hands on hips and legs in a wide stance.

What do you think happened to testosterone levels in the first posture (legs crossed, head down)?

What do you think happened to testosterone levels in the second posture (wide stance, hands on hips)?

With the legs crossed, head down posture, testosterone went down, and in the hands on hips, wide stance posture, testosterone went up.

This is because the legs crossed, head down posture signalled submission to the brain, which lowered testosterone. Lowered testosterone in turn lowers motivation and ability to attack. On the other hand, the wide leg stance and the hands on the hips sends signals that we are dominant to the brain, which raises our testosterone levels making us feel more confident, energised and even ready to fight.

> *So just by changing the position of our body, we are actually having an impact on our hormones.*

Imagine the posture of somebody who is experiencing depression. It is usually head down, eyes down, a complete lack of energy. It is thought that depression may be connected to this submissive strategy and may even in some cases be a way of taking people out of situations where there is potential threat. This may keep us safe in the short term, but as we experienced just briefly in the first experiment, when we hang down, we cannot see those around us – even those who may be signalling helpful, encouraging faces. So, depression may take us away from threat, but can also, over time, take us away from sources of help (including ourselves).

The self-critic and its relationship to the dominant-submissive strategy

We will see later when we are thinking in more detail about the self-critic, that our own self-critic triggers off this dominant-submissive strategy. It has a dominant manner which can then set off a submissive strategy within us. So just talking to ourselves in a self-critical way can suddenly end up making us feel anxious, beaten down, and lacking in energy. Even depressed, and sometimes suicidal. It can be really eye-opening to discover just how fast and powerful this stimulus and response is within us. So, if we have dominance as one strategy and submission as its reciprocal strategy, we can end up just flipping between the two in our relationships with others and with ourselves. But there is another strategy which will give us an alternative to this dominant-submissive 'dance'. This is the compassionate mind and the body posture that goes with it, which now sends in a whole different set of signals: this time of confidence, support, courage, strength and safeness. The recipient, whether that is someone else or oneself, is much more likely to then be switched into a different reciprocal response: one of comfort, settling, reassurance, calming, ability to better understand the minds of others and to problem-solve, more thoughtful and so on.

Our posture as a way of keeping ourselves safe

During the hanging down/standing up exercise, sometimes people prefer the hanging down posture. When they stand up, they may feel too exposed. This can be because we are feeling a little more vulnerable at this time or may be because of longer-term experiences where we have learned to keep ourselves small and quiet to be safe. It is important to take note of how we feel in our bodies and to take this into account as we do these practices. We are learning the benefit of an upright, open, confident, steady and stable posture, but we need to take this slowly, step by step, opening ourselves up in a way that pushes us a little but not so much that we move into threat.

Just like we would with our baby – we encourage them in a new skill that will be important in their life but we 'scaffold' them by helping them, so they stretch their ability but don't feel overwhelmed and give up.

'Window of tolerance' – pushing ourselves, but not too much

The sweet spot or area in between 'too difficult' and 'not difficult enough' is sometimes called 'the window of tolerance'. We will be aiming to keep ourselves in this window as we do our practices.

- 'Too difficult' and we feel anxious, overwhelmed, frustrated and can find it hard to think.
- Not difficult enough and we can feel bored, lethargic, drowsy and switched off.
- In the middle is the place where we feel energised, perhaps a little anxious because we are pushing ourselves into new areas, but we are willing to have a go.
- In terms of our three systems, when we are at the top end of our window of tolerance, we probably have the soothing/safeness and drive systems activated, and perhaps a little bit of the threat system activated too.

You might hear people say 'get into your power pose' before you are about to do something difficult, so you feel confident rather than anxious. What people usually mean by the 'power pose' is actually a dominant posture. This would then throw us and people we are interacting with into the dominant-submissive threat-focused dynamic. When we are moving into our compassionate mind, we don't want the submissive or dominant posture. Instead, we want this place in the middle: a confident, steady, open, stable posture.

Confident body posture

Now standing up once again, stand with your feet together. Imagine being pushed by somebody (or actually try this if you are doing this with others). What happens to you?

Now imagine that they are going to push you again, how do you get ready for this?

In the first part when you were pushed, you probably wobbled over. In the second part when you got prepared for another push you probably moved your feet so that they were hip width apart. Your knees were probably also bent and springy so you could absorb the push and then stand back upright again. You may recognise this as a common stance in yoga or the martial arts where you need stability but also flexibility. This is the same principle as tall buildings built in earthquake zones, which are built with deep foundations but also with the ability to sway a little. The same with ancient trees that have withstood gales over many hundreds of years by having deep, wide roots but also the ability to sway in the wind.

Think about a baby learning to walk. They have a wide-legged stance to give themselves a broad base. As they become more skilled and confident they can narrow their base but still the steadiest base will be hip width apart.

Copying your baby's posture

Copy your baby's posture when they are in different emotional states (or imagine doing this), e.g. when they are excited, frustrated, anxious, sad, calm and curious. Note how when you embody their posture this can affect your mood too. Our posture is so powerful that changing the position of our body in relation to itself, has an impact on our mood, our thoughts, our energy level, our motivation, and even, as we will see later, the images that pop into our mind and the memories that we have easy access to.

What did you notice?

____

____

____

Even if we don't feel like it, we can shift our body into a confident, stable, steady posture and see what happens.

Even if we don't feel like it, we can shift our body into a confident, stable, steady posture and change our mood, energy, motivation, thoughts, memories, images . . .

In other words we can:

'Change our body to change our mind.'

(Professor Paul Gilbert)

Your reflections and notes on this section about posture.

What do you want to hold onto and take forward?

____

____

____

____

____

____

So now, sitting down, with your feet hip width apart, sitting back in your chair feeling fully supported, feet flat on the floor, back upright, shoulders back and down, head upright and facing forward, we are ready to move into stepping stone two; the breath.

Module 11: The five stepping stones from threat to soothing and safeness: 2) The breath

A lot was covered in the section on posture, but we can bring it all together within just a minute or so. With each practice, including this one about the breath, we will start with posture first.

Practice: Posture and breath

- Take a seat, sitting back in the chair so you feel fully supported, but with your feet able to be firmly flat on the floor. Put something under your feet if you are not able to reach the floor when you sit back in the chair. (Or you can do this standing up, and in fact it will be important to practise this standing up at some point and then walking around, in order to really embody this confident posture as you go about your life.)
- Place your feet hip width apart. Spread your toes and find the maximum contact your feet can make with the ground (this is easier with bare feet).
- Close your eyes or find something to rest your eyes on so that you can focus inwards on your body more easily.
- Imagine a feeling of warmth or energy coming up from the ground into the soles of your feet. Imagine it moving up your legs, into the base of your spine, then moving up your spine. Imagine your spine unfurling like a fern in the spring. Bring your shoulders up to your ears, drop them back, and drop them down. Notice the feeling of openness and space in your chest.
- Slow down your in breath. Notice the pause between in and out breath, then allow your out breath to flow out of your body, from the base of your lungs all the way out of your body.

- It can sometimes help to rest your hand on your belly or chest to feel the gentle rhythm of your breath. Imagine breathing all the way down into your belly.
- On your next out breath, in your mind it can help to say very slowly, 'breath, slowing, down'.
- Then on your next out breath, in your mind it can help to say very slowly, 'body, slowing, down'.
- It can sometimes help to imagine something like sitting watching a candle flame moving back and forth in time with your slow, gentle in and out breath, or watching ripples and then stillness on a mountain lake in the breeze, or just watching a gentle wave on a beach moving up the beach with your in breath, and then slowly moving down the beach with your out breath. Whatever helps to begin to slow your breathing down.
- If it feels hard to focus on your breath, try slowly tracing up your fingers as you breath in and down them as you breath out, or tracing slowly round the pattern on a tennis ball for example.
- Your breath will begin to settle into its own soothing rhythm, usually with the out breath longer than the in breath, but at least the same length as each other.
- Your breathing is smooth, deep and regular.
- You might notice that your body is beginning to feel more settled, more stable, a little steadier.

End of practice.

This breath is very calming on its own, and is a very powerful way of settling ourselves if we feel anxious.

> *Slow, smooth, steady breathing is very calming.*
>
> *Even used on its own, it is a very powerful way of calming and settling ourselves if we feel anxious, stirred up or overwhelmed.*
>
> *And we always have it with us wherever we go.*

Tips: If it's hard to make the out breath longer than the in breath

- **Seven eleven breathing**

Breathe in for seven seconds then out for eleven seconds. Counting can help to externalise focus away from the body.

- **Ocean breathing**
    - Sit upright as if in a 'dignified' manner.
    - Pull the stomach in to expand the rib cage to help to breathe deeper and slower.
    - Breathe in through nose, placing the tongue gently on the roof of mouth behind the top teeth.
    - Constrict the throat as if trying to fog a mirror but with mouth closed and breathe out, slowly making the sound of the ocean.

This type of breathing can really help to extend the out breath much more than we might normally be able to. It can be very calming.

- **Square breathing – 4,4,4,4**

Breathe in for a count of four, pause on the in breath for a count of four, breathe out for a count of four, pause on the out breath for a count of four (imagine moving round the sides of a square for each part).

The focus on the pause between the in and the out breath can help to increase the out breath and slow the whole breathing rhythm down.

- **Mobile phone or computer apps**

There are many apps to help with the rhythm of your breathing, including some which use wonderful visualisations, for example following the opening and closing of a flower.

- **Toning**

Toning is making a deep, resonant 'hum' or 'mmmmm' or long 'ou' sound as in 'you'. First breathe in deeply all the way to the base of your lungs then make your toning sound, deeply and slowly on your out breath. Notice the feeling of the vibration of the sound.

This method really helps the deepening of the out breath and takes the focus away from the breath and on to the sound and the feeling of the vibration. It can be very calming for yourself and also for your baby if you hold them to your chest while you do this.

Humming, using resonant and deep-sounding musical instruments, and the use of chanting and sounds in meditation is worldwide. This is a very natural and indeed ancient way of feeling calm.

Humming and using a one-stringed instrument have been found to be calming to babies in neonatal units, particularly when talking and singing is too stimulating for them.

Toning can be a really good way of intercepting high anxiety and panic when slow breathing isn't working for you or is hard to do.

It can be worth finding videos or music online by searching for 'vocal toning meditation' or 'vocal humming meditation' so you can practise, learn, and then remember the feeling in your body.

- **'Milkshake' breathing**

Imagine you have a full glass of your favourite milkshake (or another drink if you'd prefer). Now imagine blowing into it slowly and gently through a straw, just strong enough to make little bubbles and not so much that the milkshake bubbles over out of the glass.

This really helps to lengthen the out breath whilst taking your attention away from the breath itself and focusing instead on the image of it. You can also try it for real and then have the body memory (where you remember the feeling in your body) of it to help you.

This is a good one to teach children but works very well for adults too.

You might notice your baby will go through a stage of blowing bubbles from their mouth. They are exploring the sound, and the sensations of it. They usually enjoy the great reaction it can get from other people too. So in terms of the three circles, it will create some green (soothing) and some interest and excitement (blue).

- **Calming the breath through activity (see below)**

Calming the breath through activity

Sometimes when we get too caught up with our breath but need to settle and calm ourselves, it can be better to take the attention away from the breath and body completely. Doing an activity which we find calming has the effect of slowing our breathing without us thinking about it.

Some ideas for calming activities (many can be done with your child):

- Colouring in children's books or free colouring
- Playing with sand
- Playing with dried rice and lentils
- Finger painting
- Put paint in a food bag, seal it and just 'smoosh' it around
- 'Backwards colouring' – drawing the outlines around coloured shapes
- Reading
- Crocheting, knitting
- Stroking the dog or something soft
- Swaying to music
- Rocking with your baby
- Singing or humming to your baby
- Dancing with your baby
- Ironing
- Weeding a small patch of the garden
- Mending something (giving your baby something to 'mend' too if old enough)
- Painting a garden fence or a wall in the house (your little one could 'help' if you don't mind the outcome too much)
- Sweeping up
- Washing up mindfully
- Bird watching
- Watching bees
- Jumping in puddles

- Listening to sleep meditations or being read a bedtime story (search on the internet)
- Walking with your baby in a sling or buggy, finding a pace that feels calming to you
- Watching the clouds
- Wrapping up warm and stargazing
- Exercises that use the large muscles such as legs and buttocks e.g. yoga, lunges, squats
- Steady jogging if you enjoy jogging
- Doing a sticker book
- Blowing bubbles
- Listening to sounds – just letting them wash over and through you

What activities do you find calming and settling? (you can add them here to look back on if you are feeling anxious or out of sorts)

What does your baby find calming and settling? (calmness can be catching – so when one or other of you is calm, it can calm the other one – even our pets can become calmer)

Your reflections and notes on this section about the breath.

What do you want to hold onto and take forward?

___

___

___

___

___

Module 12: The five stepping stones from threat to soothing and safeness: 3) Facial expression and 4) Voice tone

Practice: Breath, posture, face and voice

- Putting stepping stones one and two together as we move into stepping stone three; sit upright in a chair, feeling fully supported by it, with your feet flat on the floor, hip width apart.
- Close your eyes or gently focus on one spot and imagine warmth or energy flowing up through the soles of your feet, up your legs, up your spine. Bring your shoulders up to your ears and then drop them back and down, feeling the expansion, openness and space in your chest.
- Slow down your in breath, breathing gently and deeply into your belly (rest your hands on your belly if you wish, to feel this rise and fall), pause, and then breathe slowly all the way out, using your ocean breathing, toning or milkshake breathing (see above) if this helps.
- You might notice your body feeling steadier and more stable as your breath slows down.
- Now bring a warm, kind smile to your face. It can help to imagine seeing someone or something that you care about in the distance, such as a pet, a beloved friend, a tree or plant that is particularly dear to you, your home, or your car for example. Whatever makes you smile when you see it or think of it.
- Notice how you feel in your body.
- Now bring a neutral expression to your face. Notice how you feel in your body.

- Now bring the warm, friendly expression to your face. Notice how that feels.
- And back to the neutral facial expression. Notice how that feels.
- Now imagine saying 'Hello' and your name with a neutral tone of voice. Notice how it feels in your body.
- Now imagine saying 'Hello' and your name with a warm, friendly voice as if you are really pleased to see yourself in the distance. How does that feel in your body?
- Now back to a neutral voice. Notice how that feels.
- Now back to greeting yourself with a warm, friendly tone of voice. Notice how that feels.
- Imagine that you are walking round a corner, and you see in the distance, yourself, with a warm face and voice, looking and sounding really pleased to see you. How does that feel in your body?
- Now imagine coming round the corner and you see yourself looking at you with a neutral face and saying 'Hello' in a neutral voice tone. How does that feel in your body?
- Choose which facial expression and voice tone you wish to bring for the rest of this practice.
- Just notice your breath, moving in and out, perhaps resting your hand on your belly.
- Shift your attention to the sounds or the silence, allowing whatever you find to come in through your ears as if your ears are satellite dishes.
- Now bring your attention to the feel of your feet on the floor, gently moving them, then the feel of the chair steady underneath you, then the feel of your hands, just moving them gently.
- Gently open your eyes.

End of practice.

What did you notice during this practice?

How did you feel?

People often comment on the impact of changing their face and voice from neutral to warm and friendly and back again. Often people find the warm friendly face and voice makes them feel physically warm, calm, and lighter (even feeling like the sun has come out in some instances). The neutral face and voice tend to make people feel heavier and a bit down in mood.

Sometimes however the warm friendly smile can feel 'fake' to people, and they mistrust it even when it's their own smile. This can happen if you feel a bit self-conscious but may reflect actual experiences you've had.

The impact of our own face and voice on ourselves is so important as they are both ways of switching on our soothing system very quickly. This is because we are social beings and are wired to feel safe when people regard us with warmth and kindness. We then 'micro-mimic' these expressions and voice tones in our own body, which then stimulates the vagus nerve (part of the parasympathetic nervous system which is stimulated by signals of social safeness such as a warm smile or voice tone) which in turn calms our breathing and our heart rate, and releases oxytocin, which gives us that 'warm' feeling.

We feel soothed and safe when people regard us and talk to us with warm, kind faces and voices.

We also feel soothed and safe when we bring a warm, kind face and voice to ourselves.

Working on bringing this warm, kind voice and face to ourselves is very powerful, and worth persisting with, even if initially it feels a little strange or uncomfortable. This can be changed through practice, even in those who find it particularly challenging. Just take it slowly, steadily, step by step.

Your reflections and notes on this section about facial expression and voice tone.

What do you want to hold onto and take forward?

____

____

____

____

____

Module 13: The five stepping stones from threat to soothing and safeness: 5) Mindfulness

We briefly looked at mindfulness at the beginning of the book. Here we are going to pull it together with all five stepping stones into the full practice that Paul Gilbert refers to as 'soothing breathing rhythm' (sometimes called 'SBR' for short). There will also be some more detailed mindfulness practices.

This first part (posture, breath, face and voice) will be familiar to you.

Practice: Bringing mindfulness into soothing breathing rhythm

- Sit in your chair, bottom right back in it so you feel fully supported, and place your feet flat on the floor, hip width apart, sitting in a 'dignified' posture which feels steady and stable.
- Sit upright, bringing your shoulders to your ears, then dropping them back and down. Notice the openness and space in your body and your steady, stable posture.
- Slow down your in breath, allowing your breath to come all the way into the base of your lungs, perhaps placing your hands on your belly to feel the rise and fall. Pause your breath for a moment. Then breathe slowly out, using ocean breathing, toning or milkshake breathing if these help. Enjoy the slow rhythm of your breath and the rise and fall of your belly.
- Bring a warm friendly facial expression, as if you have just seen someone or something that you're really delighted to see in the distance. Imagine greeting them or it with warmth and delight; 'Hello!'
- Now bring your warm kind face and voice to your breath, just noticing without judgement how it feels to breathe in, wherever you notice it. Perhaps your nose, your throat, your belly. Notice the pause, and then notice the out breath – breathing all the way out.

End of practice.

We can bring this warm, kind observation or mindfulness to any aspect of this practice – the thoughts that come and go in our mind, physical sensations in our body, memories that arise and fade away, sounds outside or inside your room – anything at all. Mindfulness in itself can be calming, but here we are also bringing with it a texture of warmth and kindness to whatever comes into our awareness. This is the basis of true mindfulness, where a deliberate and conscious awareness is coupled with a motivation to be compassionate to whatever we find appearing in that awareness.

Practice: Two-minute soothing breathing rhythm

- Sit or stand with feet flat on the floor, hip width apart.
- Bring your shoulders up, back and down so you feel open, steady and stable (*'body like a mountain'*).
- Bring a warm, friendly smile to your face, and hear your warm friendly voice, perhaps saying 'Hello' to you.
- Bring your warm, kind attention to your breath. Slow down your in breath, pause, and then slowly breathe out, perhaps making the humming or ocean sound.
- Just enjoy for a moment the feel of your breath slowing down, and with it your body slowing down, becoming steadier, and more stable (*'breath like the wind'*).
- Just observe your mind, your feelings, your body for a moment from the slight distance that mindfulness brings, rather than feeling swept away and caught up in them (*'mind like the sky'* – focusing on the blue of the sky rather than the clouds that move across it).
- Now set off from here to whatever is next but from this mind and body of calm and steadiness.

End of practice.

This expression from Buddhism along with the addition of face and voice can be a helpful way of remembering all five stepping stones.

'Body like a mountain, breath like the wind, mind like the sky.'

All with a warm, kind, face and voice.

More mindfulness practices

Mindfulness has been found to have many benefits to both mother and baby in terms of physical and psychological health during pregnancy, birth and after birth. It allows us to 'unhook' ourselves from our thoughts, sensations, emotions and so on, so that rather than getting carried along by them without realising it, and getting caught in our reactions to them, we can let them come and go without responding to them. It also enables us to become better at identifying what needs action. We can more accurately tune into what is happening and notice changes that we might not expect. We can also see that what our threat system might decide is fixed and unchangeable, is actually variable and more nuanced. It opens the possibility that what we assume is the case, may actually not be. This is particularly important if our threat brain gets hold of us, because it is designed to make fast decisions which err on the side of caution. This means we often end up staying in threat unnecessarily.

Practising mindfulness literally changes our brain. So, the more we do, the more we are becoming different in how we process information and manage ourselves and the world around us, including how we are with our baby.

Practice: Mindfulness to sounds

This can be a good starting practice when you are exploring mindfulness.

- Sit upright with your eyes closed or gently focused on an object, in your 'dignified' posture, with your back and head upright, feet hip width apart and flat on the floor so that you feel grounded and steady. Bring your shoulders up to your ears, then drop them back and down, noticing the increase in sense of space in your body.

- Bring your warm, kind face and voice to yourself, perhaps saying hello to yourself with real warmth – ('Hello . . . !'). Allow your breathing to begin to slow and settle, finding its own slow, smooth, soothing rhythm.
- *'Body like a mountain, mind like the sky, breathe like the wind'*
- Now begin to tune into the sounds around you. Imagine your ears are like satellite dishes that allow in all the sounds.
- When your mind wanders away, just gently guide it back to sounds, like you might guide a young child or puppy that has wandered away. This wandering is what our minds are designed to do. Each time you notice it has wandered off is a moment of mindfulness. The more you notice and return, the more you are building the wiring in your brain for mindful focusing.
- You might notice that sometimes you focus on sounds in the room, and sometimes outside the room, sometimes sounds from your body. Sometimes you may not detect any sound at all. Just notice it just as it is.
- You may find you have a reaction to certain sounds. Perhaps they startle you or annoy you. Or you may enjoy them and not want them to end. Just notice your reaction in the same mindful manner – with warm curiosity, allowing the reactions to be just as they are. Then shift your mind once again to the sounds coming in through your ears.
- Sit for as long as you can.
- Try sitting beyond the point at which you have decided 'That is enough'. There is a lot to be learned from riding through the point at which you would ordinarily have finished. It allows you to explore the discomfort, your ability to bear it and to find that it is often possible to get back into that state of calm mindfulness once again. This is very helpful to be able to tuck away into our knowledge about ourselves.
- When you are ready, move your attention to the feel of your chair supporting you, your feet in contact with the floor, and the feel of your hands. Perhaps moving them. Then open your eyes. You may want to stretch and move. See if you can carry this calm, centred state with you into the next part of your day.

End of practice.

Your reflections about this practice. What would you like to hold onto and remember from this practice?

Practice: Mindfulness to your cup of tea (or whatever drink you like)

- Sit in your dignified posture ('body like a mountain' or mighty oak tree), feet hip width apart and in contact with the floor. Your back and head are upright. Bring your shoulders up to your ears and drop them back and down, feeling the space opening up in your body.
- Bring your warm, kind, face, and warm, kind voice to yourself in this practice, welcoming yourself here. Perhaps in your mind you say 'Hello [your name].' Bring this same warmth and welcoming to your breath, allowing your breath to begin to slow and settle into its soothing rhythm.
- Take hold of your cup of tea (or whatever drink you choose). Notice the temperature of your cup, the feel of the texture of the cup, the weight of the cup, how it feels where it meets your hands.
- Notice the appearance of your cup and the light and the shade on the cup. Notice how the liquid looks inside of the cup – any reflections, and variations in colour. Notice how it moves as you move the cup.
- Become aware of any sounds or no sounds as you move the cup.
- Allow the smells from your drink to come into your nose. Hold your reaction with the same calm, mindful attention, just noticing your reaction without needing it to be any different. Notice any other smells, perhaps more subtle smells or other smells in the air.
- Take a sip and hold the drink in your mouth. Notice the feel of the liquid in your mouth – the temperature of it, the texture of it, how it moves in your mouth. Notice any changes in taste as it spreads across your tongue. Notice the feel of the liquid on your lips.

- Notice any urges to swallow it or to dry or lick your lips. Notice just what these urges feel like – how do you know that you want to swallow – what tells you this?
- Then swallow the liquid whilst paying attention to the feeling of swallowing. Notice any sensations or tastes that are left behind.
- See if you can take a few more sips in this manner.
- When you are ready, shift your attention to the feel of the chair supporting you. Feel your feet and your hands, perhaps moving them. When you are ready, gently open your eyes and look around the room. See if you can keep hold of this state of calm mindfulness as you move into the next part of your day.

End of practice.

Reflections on this practice. What did you notice? What would you like to hold onto and remember from this?

____

____

____

This practice can give us some insight into the wonder our baby experiences many times a day as they encounter new things. We can see what it is like to really immerse ourselves in our experiences like our baby does, and to see what is new in what we thought we knew really well.

Practice: Mindfulness to my baby asleep on me

- Bring your warm, kind face and warm, kind voice to this practice, perhaps saying a gentle 'Hello!' to yourself and your baby.
- Bring your warm attention to your breath and allow your breathing to slow down. Just feel the rhythm of your breath. As it finds its own soothing rhythm, you might notice a feeling of groundedness and steadiness.
- Notice what supports you – what is holding you up? – perhaps a chair, sofa or bed. Notice how it feels to be held and supported in this way. Notice the feel of your body in contact with it.
- Bring your attention to the feel of your baby on you. What do you notice?
- (You might feel the weight of them on you, the feel of where their body makes contact with yours. You might feel the warmth of their body against yours.)
- Notice the movements your baby makes, the gentle rhythm of their breath, any fluttering of the eyes behind their eyelids, movements of their mouth, and expressions on their face. There may be movements of hands, of fingers, of arms and legs.
- Notice the texture of your baby's skin, perhaps gently stroking it, noticing how it feels under your fingers. You might notice the variations in colour and pattern.
- Shift your attention to how your baby's body moves with the gentle rhythm of your breathing and as you move positions.
- Notice how you feel inside to be sitting with your baby in this moment. Allow whatever you feel to be here; it might be joy, contentment, relief, irritation, frustration . . . Just bring your mindful attention of warmth, curiosity, acceptance and allowing. Notice whether this feeling stays exactly as it is or whether it shifts and changes like clouds moving across a sky.
- Bring your attention to smells. Perhaps breathe in the smell of your baby, or the intermingling of the smell of you and your baby. Notice any other smells. Become aware of any changes in the intensity of what you smell, the variability in the smells.

- Notice the sounds. Perhaps the tiny sounds of your baby's breathing. Perhaps the sounds of your breathing. The gurgling of your stomach, the sound of your clothes against your chair or whatever you are sitting on as you move. You might notice other sounds in the room or outside of the room. Become aware of any reactions to them and allow those reactions to be held loosely, without judgement, just allowing them to come and go.
- Notice any thoughts coming into your mind. Allow them to float in and out of your mind like clouds moving across the sky.
- Allow your attention to take in the whole picture of you here with your baby. See if there is anything else you notice from this perspective. Just allow whatever you notice to arise, notice it loosely, then allow it to float away.
- When you are ready to finish, see what it might be like to thank yourself and your baby for this experience together.

End of practice.

Your reflections about this practice. What did you notice? What would you like to hold onto and remember from this practice?

____

____

____

Putting soothing breathing rhythm ('the five stepping stones from threat to soothing') into practice

The times we usually need soothing breathing rhythm (SBR) are generally when we feel very anxious, cross or stirred up. In other words when we are in our threat system. The trouble is when we are in our threat system, we often don't even think of how we can switch out of it into a more settled and calm state (see the chapter about 'multiple selves' for more on this). Instead, we tend to get pulled into more angry or anxiety-provoking thoughts and behaviours (like when we are late for something and our child refuses to get dressed and we just end up feeling more panicked and angry). This is just the nature of our human brain and body.

We need to therefore practise SBR when things are easy, such as when we are calm, when we have a bit of time, in other words, when we don't particularly need it. But by practising it, the brain and the body learn it and it becomes easier and easier, firstly to remember to do it, and secondly to develop a fast track to the feeling of calmness. It's like going to a place that makes you feel settled and happy which then creates a memory. You then don't need to physically go there to feel settled and happy, just remembering it changes your body and mind. You have a short cut.

Like anything, you might need reminders to practise. Here are some ideas:

Ideas to help you remember to practise

- Put an hourly sound on your phone which reminds you to do the practice, whatever activity you are doing (if possible).
- Put sticky notes or little smiley face stickers, for example, in key places, e.g. on the handle of the buggy, where you first look in the morning, next to the kettle, on the car steering wheel, on the nappy changing mat, on the washing-up liquid bottle.
- Assign a particular time for practice which you do every day, e.g. while you wash your face in the morning, when you make your first cup of tea of the morning, when your baby is having a nap – whatever works for you.

Does soothing breathing rhythm make a difference?

For us to commit to something, especially something as difficult as trying to switch from threat to soothing, we need to be convinced that it is worth the effort. And it doesn't usually help if someone just tells us; we need to have experienced it for ourselves.

One way which can be helpful is to engage in something after doing SBR, then another time do it without SBR and see what the difference might be.

Here are some ideas for when you could try SBR and then try the activity in your usual way:

- Going to pick up your baby from their cot
- Feeding your baby
- Just before you clean your teeth or take a shower
- Before putting on face cream or body lotion
- Whilst walking with the buggy
- Before you start your car

The aim of this list is to put SBR to the test on things that are not too challenging; however, some of those listed above may be very challenging for you. If so, write your own list here of when it would be easiest to try out SBR before an activity:

My list of easy activities that I will use to test the difference between doing SBR and not doing SBR before I start them:

____

____

____

____

____

Then you could try using it in slightly more challenging situations, for example:

- Before making a phone call that you are a bit worried about

- Changing your baby when they are a bit unhappy
- Getting up to start the dinner when you feel tired
- Going out with your baby when you are not really feeling like it
- When you are trying to think of ideas for dinner

Again, this list will be personal to you. The idea is to be able to bring a different body and mind to whatever you are going to do, to see if it makes a difference. The more you try this, the clearer it will become and the easier it will be to draw on it in the future, particularly when things are more difficult.

My list of slightly more difficult activities that I want to see if SBR makes a difference to:

____

____

____

____

____

The hope is of course that it does make a difference to you and that you find it helpful. But it might be that it needs tweaking, or practice, or you may find your own way of switching systems. We will look at lots more ideas in this book and take it step by step.

Your reflections and notes on this section about mindfulness and soothing breathing rhythm.

What do you want to hold onto and take forward?

____

____

____

____

____

Module 14: Uncertainty: The place between threat and soothing

We have so far discussed the threat system and its antidote, the soothing/safeness system. However, there is another, much less talked about system or state that exists between them both. This is the state of uncertainty. This occurs when our sense of what keeps us feeling safe becomes less certain or starts to disappear. Our threat system then begins to be released from the 'brake' of the soothing/safeness system. If you imagine those little pull-back toy cars that are ready to speed off the moment you lift your hand off them, or the dog pulling on their lead, who races off if you let go of the lead, the soothing/safeness system acts as the 'hand', 'lead', or the 'brake' on the threat system.

What this means is that we can begin to experience the sensations of being in threat, such as a racing heart, a churning stomach or worrying thoughts, *even when there is no threat*. People might experience this as chronic anxiety or constant worry, even when there seems to be nothing to worry about. Although no threat is present, safeness has been lost or is becoming less certain.

> *We can begin to experience the sensations of being in threat, such as a racing heart, a churning stomach or worrying thoughts,*
>
> *even when there is no threat.*

These are some examples that people have given of where they begin to feel anxious even in the absence of threat, where instead safeness has become less certain:

- When the midwife leaves the room during the birthing process even though all is still going well and nothing much is happening.
- When your partner returns to work or your mother returns home after you've had your baby even though you feel confident with the baby.
- When a parent becomes ill or their car is out of action so they can't come over to help you, even though you don't need them at the moment.

- When you run low on a particular food or other item (e.g. toilet rolls) even though you know it will easily last until the next shop.
- When you or your partner get a minor illness.
- When you sleep elsewhere without your normal pillow.
- When you try to sleep without a sheet over your back during hot weather.

What are some of your examples of where you begin to feel anxious through loss or uncertainty about safeness, even in the absence of threat?

____

____

____

____

Your baby will be highly attuned to uncertainty as the stakes are so much higher for them. Examples for them might be:

- Trying to sleep in a light sleepsuit when they are used to a heavier one.
- When you begin to leave the room even though they were quite happy doing what they were doing.
- When they lose their favourite comforter even though nothing threatening is happening.
- When you take your hand off them even though they appeared sound asleep.
- When a routine is slightly different e.g. the other parent to usual reads them their bedtime book, or a different towel to usual being used at bathtime.

What are some examples of uncertainty for your baby?

____

____

It seems that the chronic stress that can result from ongoing uncertainty can cause both psychological and physical health problems. It may be one of the missing links between early childhood adversity and the chronic health problems that have been documented, such as obesity, irritable bowel syndrome, diabetes, cancer, stroke and so on. One hypothesis is that the chronic stress caused by uncertainty creates a chronic inflammatory response in our body which then leads to many of these diseases.

In a kind of 'chicken and egg' scenario; our internal body and brain systems are constantly monitoring us physically for signs of less certainty around our health. This means that we can even begin to feel uneasy because our brain has identified changes in our body that we are not consciously aware of. When we do become physically or mentally unwell, even if it is not serious, we can feel a degree of anxiety or of feeling out of balance, or 'up ended' which seems out of proportion to the illness. This is because our brain is registering that our body is not as robust as usual. This is why becoming less fit, or more fragile with age, can be linked with chronic anxiety.

Uncertainty has also been identified as a risk factor in perinatal mental illness, linked to aspects such as uncertainty with regard to social support.

Some interesting studies have shown that when we can have certainty, for example around our partner being able to take leave whenever it's needed for a certain period of time after the baby is born, then there is a reduction in physical and mental health problems in the postnatal period including mastitis, hospital stays, antibiotic and antidepressant use.

This is therefore such a crucial area, particularly it seems in times such as the perinatal period.

Rather than dismissing chronic anxiety and worry as 'you are just creating something to worry about', or 'you worry for worry's sake', we can now look to see not just what the threat might be, but whether there has been a loss of, or uncertainty about, safeness.

How might your compassionate mind help you when you are feeling anxiety due to uncertainty? (Remember that it is the soothing/safeness system beginning to loosen or disappear that is the issue – so practices that re-stimulate the soothing/safeness system will help to settle you again, or certainly enable you to reach out to begin accessing safeness once more, perhaps from other people or from your environment.)

____

____

____

____

Here are some examples that others have found helpful:

- It can be enough just to realise that, for example, your partner's return to work has caused this increase in anxiety.
- Perhaps take steps to increase the sense of certainty, e.g. knowing that your partner will call you every lunchtime or that they have agreed with their boss that you may need to call at any point over the next few months.
- Have a series of backups in place, or develop an 'if this, then this' plan about anything that is worrying you.
- Practise something step by step to build your confidence.
- Prioritise your mental and physical health and recovery after childbirth so that your internal systems register safeness rather than uncertainty.
- Do regular compassionate mind practices to keep stimulating the soothing/safeness system.

Your reflections and notes on this section about uncertainty in relation to threat and safeness/soothing.

What do you want to hold onto and remember? What would you like to take forward?

____

____

____

____

____

Module 15: How the soothing/safeness system relates to compassion

There is sometimes an understandable assumption that the green system of soothing and safeness is the compassion system. If we go back to the idea of the old brain and the new brain, then the green system is the part of the old brain used primarily for resting and digesting. A key part of the soothing system in many animals is also the motivation to be cared for and to be caring. Our baby has a soothing/safeness system, so they want to be cared for, and when they are cared for, it makes them feel soothed and safe. But we wouldn't see them as able to choose to be caring when they are very young, or to be compassionate. (Although they do have an early sense of right and wrong, fairness and helpfulness at a surprisingly young age, which has led researchers to see compassion as innate rather than something we have to learn from scratch. Though of course we can learn it too, hence this book.) We can also see that our dog, cat or pet hamster enjoys feeling safe and soothed but again they are not capable of being compassionate because they do not have our new brain capabilities of understanding the minds of others, and then intentionally choosing how best to help a particular person. Dog owners may beg to differ here, as dogs are very sensitive to distress in their owners and come to lick them and sit with them. But do they have a mind that can decide intentionally to be caring and then work out just how to help this particular person in this moment? People may argue that they do.

These are the attributes of compassion as defined by Paul Gilbert:

- A motivation to be caring, helpful and not harmful.
- Ability to be sensitive to suffering.
- Sympathy – being able to feel moved about the suffering.
- Distress tolerance – ability to be able to bear the feelings that arise in ourselves and others.
- Empathy – to understand that what we might find helpful might be different to what someone else might find helpful in the same scenario.
- Non-judgement – to be able to hold what arises in ourselves and others without criticising or judging it.

Compassion also requires action to try to prevent or alleviate that suffering, which might be compassionate behaviour, compassionate thinking, using compassionate imagery and so on, which we will look at in detail throughout this book.

So, compassion requires abilities from our old brain (a motivation to be caring) and from our new brain (empathy, non-judgement, etc). Perhaps our dog can do many of these aspects, and even those that we find difficult, but they would struggle with new brain aspects such as empathy – really being able to put themselves in our shoes.

When we struggle to be compassionate to ourselves or to others, there can be many reasons for this, some of which we will cover in this book, but it can be helpful to come back to this list of attributes to see if there are particular ones that we struggle with, e.g. tolerating distress. Once we identify what is more difficult for us, we can focus more precisely on firstly being compassionate to the fact we struggle with this, as this will not be our fault, and then secondly, set about trying to help ourselves or finding help for this specific issue.

Looking through the list of attributes above, which do you find the hardest?

____

____

____

____

Are there times when you find some easier and some harder? (When we are exhausted, hungry, pressured for time, overwhelmed, for example, we find aspects of compassion, and compassion in general, much more difficult – this is not our fault.)

____

____

____

____

Are there some attributes that you struggle with generally?

___

___

___

___

We all have differences within us, for example, due to brain injury, neurological differences such as autism or attention deficit hyperactivity disorder (ADHD), our upbringing and experiences, which generally shape the way our brain works and can impact giving or receiving compassion. Again, these are not our fault. The more we understand about ourselves the more we can work with and around these aspects to enable us to be as helpful as possible to ourselves and others, within our limits and in expanding our limits.

So, if compassion and soothing are not the same thing, then how do they relate to each other? In order to be compassionate, we need to be able to set off from a system that has been switched from threat to soothing. If we stay in threat, then it would be very difficult to access all those attributes listed above as the motivational system to be caring and to accept care sits in the old brain soothing system and this is the system that underpins our motivation to be compassionate. If we stayed in the threat system then the kind of motivations that would arise would be things like 'attack', 'hide from' or 'compete with', rather than 'care for'.

Not only does the caring system sit in the soothing system, but when we do switch into the soothing/safeness system, this gives us the best chance of accessing the part of our brain that is to do with understanding the minds of others (needed for empathy), being able to look out with a wide focus (required for the ability to notice suffering in ourselves and others), sympathy, distress tolerance and non-judgement.

> So, to give ourselves the best chance to be able to give and receive compassion we need to switch systems from threat to soothing first.

Compassion in relation to soothing can be represented like this:

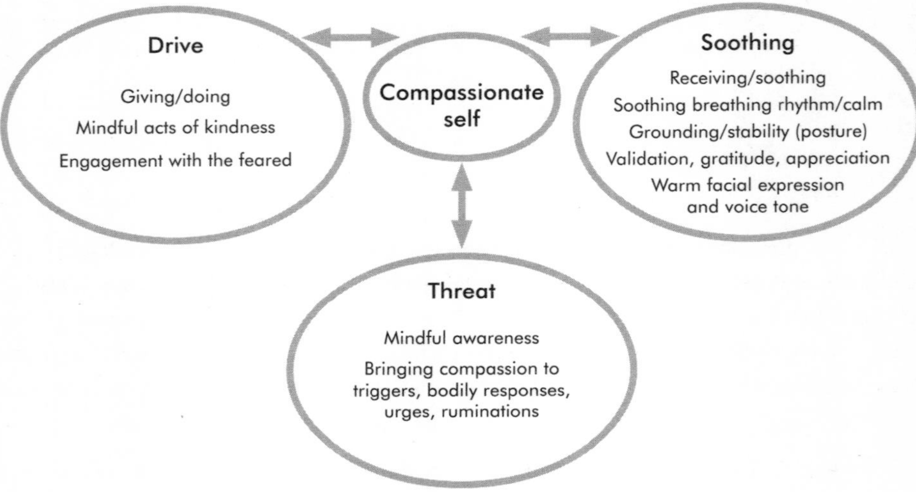

Figure 6: The compassion process
Reproduced with kind permission of Paul Gilbert.

In this diagram we can see that we use our soothing system to change our body, which then changes how we think, which then helps us to move into our compassionate mind in order to approach our threat and drive systems from an intention to be helpful. Of course, the whole intention and decision to move to our soothing system to aid our compassionate motivation in itself comes from a compassionate motivation. So it is rather 'chicken and egg'. The more we understand about the power of compassion and practise it, the easier it is when we are in threat to remember that compassion is helpful. This helps us to pause and try to switch systems from threat to soothing, so that we can then return to what has triggered our threat system, but now from a position of compassion.

> One way somebody used to remember this process was to imagine that when she was angry, anxious, sad or self-critical, she needed to find the 'ladder' that enabled her to climb up to her compassionate self. Each rung was one of the stepping stones from threat to soothing (posture, breath, kind face, kind voice, mindfulness). Once she reached her compassionate mind, she then turned and looked down to be with and help her angry, anxious, sad or self-critical part using her compassionate mind.

Your reflections and notes on this section about how the soothing/safeness system relates to compassion.

What do you want to hold onto and remember? What would you like to take forward?

Section 3:

Developing our compassionate mind

Module 16: The use of imagery to develop our compassionate mind

The aim of the compassion-focused approach is to stimulate the feeling of safeness, soothing and settling within us because it has so many powerful effects on us and on the people around us, including our baby.

We can stimulate this feeling in many ways, including what we focus our attention on, how we think, the particular memories we focus on, the behaviour we engage in and so on. Another way is by generating images that make us feel safe.

Think about going out to your favourite place to get something to eat. You are eating a bit later than usual, so you are hungry. What happens in your body when you look at the menu and see and smell the food that other people are eating?

____

____

____

(Your stomach might start rumbling and you might get an increase in saliva in your mouth.)

What happens if you *imagine* some delicious food?

____

____

____

Even when the food is not real, we still experience actual physical responses in our body.

What happens in your body if you see someone you fancy on the TV or in a film?

____

____

____

(You might feel a bit hot; your heart might speed up; you might experience symptoms of arousal.)

What happens in your body if you *imagine* seeing that person you fancy?

____

____

____

Again, we experience the same physical responses in our body, even though this is just in our mind. And of course, sexual fantasy is a very common way to give us some useful physical 'help' when our relationship has lost its original sparkle.

How do you feel in your body when somebody is harsh and critical of you?

____

____

____

(You might feel sick, anxious, angry, collapsed, with your heart beating fast.)

How do you feel in your body if you *imagine* somebody being harsh and critical of you?

____

____

____

Again, you might feel just the same as if it really happened. Indeed, this can be the source of our 'What if?' e.g. 'What if I upset them?' We can imagine just how they might be towards us, and how we might feel. And of course, those of us with a self-critic really do live with this imaginary critic inside of us which leaves us feeling the same as if an actual person was criticising us. (See the chapter about working with the self-critic for more about this.)

How do you feel when somebody is kind, warm and caring towards you?

____

____

____

(You might feel safe and soothed in your body.)

How might you feel if you imagined someone being kind, warm and caring towards you?

____

____

____

You can probably see where this is going – you would have the same physiological response of safeness and soothing. We can see that our body is as powerfully affected by our imagination as it is by reality. Both real and imagined relationships use the same systems within us. We can therefore make use of this, and deliberately create and use images of being related to with kindness, warmth and compassion to generate the same effect in our body and mind. So even if we can't access a real compassionate person when we need them, we can still bring up an imaginary one within us – and we will see just what an impact our imaginary compassionate figures can have on us.

Another quicker away of experiencing the power of imagery is the following short experiment:

Lemon experiment

- Close your eyes, hold out your hand, or imagine holding out your hand.
- Imagine a whole lemon is placed in your hand.
- Feel your hand respond to the weight of it. Feel the temperature of its skin. Notice the feel of its waxy, slightly rough skin.
- Look closely at the colour of it, and variations in texture and shape as you move it around in your hand.
- Smell the skin.
- Imagine placing it down on a chopping board and then cutting it in half. Notice the feel of cutting it, the juice on the cut piece, the shapes and colours of the cut surface.
- Now imagine bringing it your nose and smelling it.
- Then imagine sticking out your tongue and licking it.

What happened?

____

____

____

Many people have such a strong reaction that they can feel the 'sharpness' of the taste inside that bit between your ears and your jaw, and actually salivate, even though there is no lemon at all. Our imagination is so incredible that it can create actual physical responses within us.

So this is why being able to create physical feelings of safeness through imagery is such a significant part of the compassionate mind approach – but there are many other techniques for creating feelings of safeness too, so don't worry if imagery is something you struggle with. (But don't throw it away completely either, just keep it loosely with you, because you may well find it comes into its own for you at a later date; and your baby may really enjoy it too when they get older.)

The more experiences we create of safeness, the more memories of safeness we store to draw upon in the future, even if the memories come from experiences we have created in our own minds. They still create new connections in our brain, helping us to feel increasingly safe, creating changes in our epigenetics, helping us to problem solve, think creatively, and understand our baby better.

Practice: Compassionate colour

This is a lovely, simple practice that is particularly good when you feel a little out of sorts, or perhaps tired or achy. It can be done quickly if you are short of time, or more slowly for a deeper experience.

- Sit with your eyes closed or focused gently on an object, in an upright 'dignified' posture, with your feet hip width apart, flat on the floor. Bring your shoulders up to your ears, then drop them back and down, feeling the space in your chest and body.
- Bring your warm, kind face, and warm, kind voice to this practice. Focus on wherever you find your breath. Perhaps imagine greeting it warmly once you find it – 'Hello breath!'
- Begin slowing down your in breath, then really slowing down your out breath, allowing it to flow slowly up from deep inside you, all the way out, noticing the pause, before breathing in again. Slow, smooth and rhythmic.
- As your breath begins to slow down you might notice your body begins to feel heavier, steadier, sturdier and more stable.
- Now imagine a coloured light or mist appearing at some distance, or near to you. You have a sense that this light or mist has deep kindness and compassion for you. It has arrived here for you. There is something comforting, helpful and settling about this light or mist.
- You might imagine it gently surrounding you like a comforting blanket or beginning to seep into you through the pores in your skin or through the top of your head or your

heart area. You feel your body begin to ease, like the sensation of achy muscles relaxing in contact with a hot water bottle, or the warm sun on your skin on a cool spring day.

- The colour or mist flows gently round your body, allowing it to ease, settle and soothe.
- It flows down your arms and into your fingers, easing them as it goes. There may be a sense of gratitude and relief from your arms and fingers which work so hard for you.
- It flows down your legs and into your feet and toes. Imagine them enjoying the sensation of accepting this ease after keeping you moving all this time.
- The colour or mist flows into your abdomen and into your womb and internal organs. You may sense their relief and gratitude to being attended to after their experiences of working for you and your baby.
- It flows into your breasts that have born milk, and into your lungs and your heart that work day and night for you. You may sense their relief and their gratitude as the light or mist flows around them.
- It flows into your head, settling and soothing it, smoothing it when it feels frazzled, allowing it calm for a while.
- It flows into your jaw, your teeth and your tongue, allowing them to be loose.
- Notice how it feels to have this flowing around and easing the whole of your body and mind.
- Stay with this as long as you wish.
- You might like to do this whilst holding your baby – imagining the coloured light or mist flowing out through your heart, your breasts or your hands and arms into your baby, sending in warmth, compassion, care, settling and soothing.
- You may imagine the coloured light or mist coming out of your hands, arms or heart and flowing into other people or wrapping gently around them. Perhaps imagine it going across towns and cities, across the countryside, spreading throughout the country. Then even across into other countries, across seas, all the way around the world, until it arrives back at you again.

- When you feel ready, begin to bring your attention to the sense of you back in your space. Notice the sounds coming in through your ears. Notice the feel of your feet on the floor; perhaps wiggling your toes and moving your feet. Notice the feel of the seat underneath you, supporting you. When you are ready, gently open your eyes. Just take in this feeling for a moment before setting off for the next part of your day. Stretch if you need to bring your energy levels back up, perhaps standing up and moving with steadiness and calmness around your room.

End of practice.

Reflection: How was this practice for you? How did it feel? What did you notice? What would you like to remember for next time?

____

____

____

____

Your reflections and notes on this section about the use of imagery to develop our compassionate mind, and the compassionate colour practice.

What do you want to hold onto and remember? What would you like to take forward?

____

____

____

____

____

Module 17: Compassionate place/safe place/your place

This practice is often a favourite for people as it can be relatively easy to do but can have real impact. This might not of course be the same for you, but it is worth coming back to this one multiple times, as it can really shift and change and grow in its helpfulness. It is known by different names.

Practice: Compassionate place/safe place/your place

- Sit with your bottom back in your seat so you feel fully supported by it, back upright, feet flat on the floor, hip width apart.
- Move your feet to feel the contact with the floor (try this with bare feet to see how this feels). Gently close your eyes or soften your gaze, focusing on an object.
- Imagine a feeling of energy or warmth coming up from the earth, through the soles of your feet, up your legs, into your spine, up your spine. Imagine your spine unfurling, bringing your shoulders up to your ears, and dropping them back and down. Feel the space and openness in your chest.
- Turn your attention to your breath; bringing your warm, kind face and warm, kind voice to it – perhaps saying 'Hello breath!' as if you are pleased to encounter it, and so grateful for all its work, keeping you going quietly in the background, day and night.
- Allow the in breath to begin to slow down. Feel the slight pause, then allow your breath to flow all the way out from the base of your lungs, using your ocean breathing or toning if this helps in lengthening your out breath.
- On your next out breath it can help to say slowly in your mind, 'breath, slowing, down'. Then on the next out breath it can help to say in your mind, 'body, slowing, down'.

- You might notice your body beginning to feel more and more steady, calm and stable.
- Now imagine that you find yourself in a place where you can breathe out, where you feel totally at ease; a place where you can be just as you need to be, a place where you feel free. This is your place, a place that is here for you.
- It may have elements of real places, but as it is imaginary, it doesn't have to make any sense at all – it can be just as you need it to be.
- Take a look round this place and see what is here. Notice what season you are in, what time of day or night it is, whether you are inside or outside. See how these change the colours, the light and the shade.
- Become aware of the feel of the air on your skin and it feels just right. Notice the feel of whatever is under your feet, and what you can touch with your hand.
- Tune in to the sounds in this place. Notice the closer sounds, the louder sounds. Then tune in to the more distant sounds, the quieter sounds.
- Notice the smells; the stronger ones, and then behind those you might detect more subtle smells.
- Tune in to the tastes in your mouth; perhaps tastes on the air, or something you have been eating or drinking.
- Notice how you interact with this place; you might be walking, sitting, lying down, running, doing cartwheels even if you've never been able to do a cartwheel before, flying, riding a horse or a motorbike, or swimming underwater – you can do anything you wish in this place.
- You might become aware that you feel like you have a deep connection to this place; that it has arrived here just for you, that you feel welcomed in by this place. It gives you a sense that it is pleased that you are here. Notice how it feels to be so welcomed, so deeply connected. Enjoy being here for as long as you want.
- When you are ready to leave, just take a note of this place, perhaps give it a name, know it in some way, so that you can come back here easily whenever you need to.

- Shift your attention to the sense of yourself here back in your room. Tune in to the sounds, allowing them to come into your ears as if your ears are satellite dishes. Feel your chair, steady underneath you. Tune in to your feet, moving them to feel their contact with the floor. Tune into your hands, moving them, feeling your fingers.
- When you are ready, gently open your eyes.

End of practice.

Reflection: How was this practice for you? How did it feel? What did you notice? What would you like to remember for next time?

____

____

____

____

Trouble-shooting compassionate place/safe place/your place

I couldn't get an image of a place.	Some people are unable to generate any imagery, or if they can, it is not very clear. What we are aiming at here is the felt sense of being at ease and of safeness, rather than a clear image.
Every time I thought about this place being safe, I came up with all sorts of threats.	This is the power of the words we use. When we think of the word 'safe', many people shift to thinking 'how do I know this place is safe?' and that moves them into the threat system. This is why many don't call this 'safe place' anymore. Instead, we can use the language of how we might feel *if we were safe* e.g. 'at ease', 'free', 'breathe out'. • What would you call this practice? ____________________________
I couldn't settle on a place that felt right.	This can be a bit like going through different ideas for where to go on holiday, or choosing paint colours, or indeed baby names. We test them against how we feel inside, until we can go, 'something like that but perhaps with a bit more of this . . . ' We might gather ideas from books or films. Our place might change if we need it to be different on this occasion.
I have just realised that my baby wasn't there and now I feel bad about that.	This is a common experience when this practice is done in perinatal groups. Imagine if your baby was with you, how would this feel? We generated an ideal place where we can feel totally at ease. We can see that even if our baby was asleep, there is often still part of us that is on alert to them waking up. Our body and mind intuitively know the place we need and that is often with no baby in it. Or if they are in it, then perhaps they are being cared for by somebody else.

I thought it was odd that this place 'welcomed me'. I can't imagine being welcomed.	Some people have sadly rarely, if ever, felt welcomed by anyone, so this part can bring up strong emotions. It can be a bit of a leap to imagine how this place could have a mind so at first it can throw people a little. See if you can allow yourself to go with this as it can be a point at which this practice can really deepen, as it is directly stimulating our social safeness system. If you can't believe it, or don't trust it, just allow it to be there anyway, perhaps loosely, in the background. Imagine flowing around it, as if you are a river around a rock, so you still experience ease, and you begin to get used to it being here, always welcoming, no matter how you react to it.

Your reflections and notes on this section about the compassionate place/safe place/your place practice.

What do you want to hold onto and remember? What would you like to take forward?

____

____

____

____

____

Module 18: Developing our compassionate self

Qualities of the compassionate mind

If we go back to Paul Gilbert's definition of compassion: '*A sensitivity to suffering within ourselves and others, with an intention to alleviate and prevent it*', we can imagine the qualities that somebody might need in order to be able to do this. They firstly need to have an intention to be helpful which switches them into that care-giving motivational system. They need to have wisdom. For example, if somebody jumped in to save a child that had fallen into a river, then realised that they themselves couldn't swim, this would demonstrate courage but a lack of wisdom. In fact, this might end up being ultimately harmful rather than helpful as now somebody needs to risk their life rescuing two people. Building the skills to be helpful might take a great deal of commitment; for example, learning how to swim. They would also need strength of character because sometimes compassion requires us to keep going when it's hard or when we really don't feel like it. They would also need courage because turning towards suffering can be incredibly difficult and sometimes scary. And wisdom without courage might mean that nothing helpful happens despite us knowing how to help.

Qualities of the compassionate mind

Strength

Courage

Wisdom

Intention and commitment to being as helpful as best we can

Practice: A memory of our intention and commitment to be helpful as best we can

- Recall a time when you had made a decision to be helpful as best you could. It might be a moment when you helped your baby or tried to help your partner or friend with something. It could be a text message you sent that you thought might help someone. It doesn't matter whether it helped as you had hoped. This is about noticing your *intention* to be helpful.
- Notice how you feel in your body when you recall this memory.
- Notice your posture – how you are holding yourself.
- You might notice how your face looks and even how your voice might sound if you spoke.
- Imagine carrying this feeling, this voice and face, this posture, and this overall sense of your courage, with you today.

End of practice.

Reflection: How was this practice for you? How did it feel? What did you notice? What would you like to remember for next time?

____

____

____

____

Practice: A memory of strength of character

- Recall a time when you found you had great strength of character, perhaps persisting in something that was hard, or trying to stand steady and firm for something you felt was important.
- Notice how you feel in your body when you recall this memory.
- Notice your posture – how you are holding yourself.
- You might notice how your face looks and even how your voice might sound if you spoke.
- Imagine carrying this feeling, this voice and face, this posture, and this overall sense of your strength, with you today.

End of practice.

Reflection: How was this practice for you? How did it feel? What did you notice? What would you like to remember for next time?

____

____

____

____

Practice: A memory of courage

- Recall a time when you had courage. It might be going into a difficult environment, making a hard phone call, telling somebody something difficult face to face, giving birth when you are worried about it, going for a medical procedure that scares you. It might be a time when you surprised yourself by your courage.
- Notice how you feel in your body when you recall this memory.
- Notice your posture – how you are holding yourself.
- You might notice how your face looks and even how your voice might sound if you spoke.
- Imagine carrying this feeling, this voice and face, this posture, and this overall sense of your courage, with you today.

End of practice.

Reflection: How was this practice for you? How did it feel? What did you notice? What would you like to remember for next time?

___

___

___

___

Practice: Noticing times of drawing on wisdom

- Notice the times in the last day when you drew on your wisdom. It might be how you responded to your baby, working out how best to solve a problem, fixing something in the house, preparing a meal, driving a car, doing a job at work, giving somebody some advice, knowing how best to help your partner.
- We develop our wisdom throughout our lives from books we read, television programmes and films, training courses we've done, our schooling, further education courses, clips we watch on the internet, family members, family friends, friends at school, people we encounter briefly, our experiences in the world.
- I used my wisdom in the last day when

____

____

____

____

____

- Notice how you feel in your body when you recall these moments.
- Notice your posture – how you are holding yourself.
- You might notice how your face looks and even how your voice might sound if you spoke.
- Imagine carrying this feeling, this voice and face, this posture, and this overall sense of your wisdom, with you today.

End of practice.

Reflection: How was this practice for you? How did it feel? What did you notice? What would you like to remember for next time?

____

____

____

____

We can draw on these experiences and pull them together into the following imagery practice known as 'compassionate self'. Even if you could not believe that you possess any of the above qualities, try this practice and see what happens. See if you can just let it wash over you and through you with a sense of looseness and ease.

Practice: Compassionate self

- Sit with your bottom back in your chair, feet flat on the floor, hip width apart, back upright, so that you feel steady, stable and fully supported. Adopt a 'dignified' posture ('body like a mountain') so you feel steady but flexible, rather than stiff.
- Move your feet a little so that you can find full contact with the floor to help you feel grounded and steady (try it with bare feet).
- Gently close your eyes or soften them whilst focusing on an object.
- Imagine a feeling of warmth or energy bubbling up through the soles of your feet, flowing up your legs, into your spine. Imagine your spine unfurling like a fern in the spring. Bring your shoulders up to your ears, drop them back and down, feeling the increase in openness and space in your body.
- Bring your warm, friendly face and voice to your breath, perhaps in your mind saying 'Hello!' to your breath as if you are really pleased to come across it and have suddenly realised with warmth and gratitude just what it has been doing for you, quietly behind the scenes, day and night.

- Allow your in breath to slow down, breathing it all the way into the base of your lungs. Notice the pause. Then allow your out breath to really slow down, perhaps using your ocean breathing (making the sound of the sea in the back of your throat with your mouth closed) or toning (a long, deep, humming noise on your out breath to help lengthen your out breath). On your next out breath it can help in your mind to say slowly, 'breath, slowing, down'. On your next out breath it can help in your mind to say slowly, 'body, slowing, down'.
- Enjoy for a moment the feeling of your breathing finding its own soothing rhythm. As it does, you might notice your body beginning to feel steadier, sturdier, more stable.
- Now imagine a part of you that is or could be compassionate. A part of you that can be deeply caring and helpful, perhaps remembering a time when you felt caring or helpful toward somebody or something. Or a time when you really wanted to be caring or helpful. A part of you that is committed to being as helpful as you can in this moment. A part of you that tries to build your skills so that you can be as helpful as possible in the future.
- Become aware of the strength and courage of this part of you, a strength and courage that might even surprise you. A strength and courage that means you have kept going with difficult things even when you found them hard, or have stepped in to doing things that are important despite feeling anxious, scared or reluctant.
- This part of you also has great wisdom, gathered up over your lifetime. Absorbed from your experiences, from things you have read, seen in films, training you have done. All the learning you have been doing over your whole life, taking in the wisdom of family, friends, neighbours, teachers or people you may have had the briefest of moments with. All the wisdom you have taken in, gained by others over generations, including your understanding here of the difficult brain we have which we didn't choose, our human nature selected for us but not by us, to stay safe and avoid threats, all of us trying to navigate being human as best we can.
- Notice how you might move as you fully step into this warm, kind, wise, strong, caring, courageous, compassionate part of you, just for this moment.

- How does your body feel? How do your arms and legs move? You might imagine that your body changes in size or shape, that you feel bigger or steadier. Notice how you move through the world. Notice the expression on your face. Imagine as you see people in the distance how you feel towards them. Notice any heartfelt wishes you might have towards them.
- You might try out the traditional loving kindness meditation, 'May you be well, may you be happy, may you live with ease', or find the words that come spontaneously into your compassionate mind.
- You might imagine a light or a colour pouring out of you towards them.
- Notice how it feels to be able to feel like this towards others or to have the intention of sending this out as best you can even if you don't quite feel it.
- Notice how it feels in your body to be inhabiting your strong, steady, wise, kind, caring compassionate mind. Allow this feeling to settle into your body.
- Stay with this as long as you wish.
- When you are ready to finish the practice shift your attention to the sense of you back in your room. Tune in to the sounds inside the room, and outside the room, just allowing them into your ears mindfully. Turn your attention to the feel of your chair supporting you, your feet steady on the floor, moving them and feeling the floor, and your hands, moving your fingers.
- You might just make an intention to carry this part with you as far as you can into whatever you do next.
- Then gently open your eyes.

End of practice.

Your reflections on the compassionate self practice

What was this practice like for you?

How did it make you feel?

Did any difficult aspects arise for you? Any fears, blocks or resistances?

How might your compassionate self or a compassionate other help you with these?

If that fear, block or resistance could be placed on a chair and you or your compassionate self could chat to it with warm curiosity, what might it tell you about its fears? When did the fear first arise? What might its fear be for you if it were to disappear and leave you, or if it went on holiday or went off for a cup of tea when you needed it? How might your compassionate self or compassionate other help it with this fear?

What else might help?

What would you like to remember from this practice?

What might you want to work on for next time?

Trouble-shooting compassionate self

I don't think I can be compassionate.	A powerful technique is to act 'as if' you are (see below for more about this). We can even imagine acting as if we were a compassionate character from TV, film or books, or someone we know – what would they do/say/feel in this situation? You can also imagine stepping into the body of your own compassionate image/other or being.
If I become compassionate, I will feel weak, and people may take advantage of me.	This fear may have come from your own experiences. If so, that is very sad, and it's not surprising that you might feel worried. The definition of compassion is all about turning towards suffering and trying as best you can to alleviate and prevent it. It takes great strength and courage, so it is the opposite to weak. The times you have been compassionate may well have taken a great deal of strength and courage. Compassion doesn't mean doing things for others without taking care of yourself. In fact, we need to start with ourselves. That might mean protecting ourselves from the harmful behaviour of others, whilst still wishing for them to be able to find a way through whatever causes them to behave as they do. We can still face people with compassion whilst also protecting ourselves. This is represented in Buddhism as one hand being held out as 'stop' and the other hand held out palm up. Interestingly, the 'stop' hand is also thought to be related to reassurance and 'have no fear', held in a more relaxed manner with fingers slightly separated and hand slightly cupped. • Try them out and see how these hand gestures feel in your body.

I feel that I am suffering so much that I don't think I have anything to give anybody else.	We will struggle to be compassionate to others if we feel exhausted and are suffering ourselves. This is the basis of the oxygen mask principle on a plane – that we give ourselves oxygen first before our children, because if we are out of action then we are of no help to them. Once we feel well and resourced then we might find we naturally turn to considering the help we might be able to give to others. Our ability to be compassionate varies according to all sorts of things. This is just how it is. We can only do our best in this moment.

When you might use compassionate self

- Getting ready to pick your baby up when they have just woken up
- Feeding your baby
- Changing your baby
- When getting everyone ready to get out of the house
- When trying to problem-solve something
- When driving your car or pushing your baby in the buggy
- When putting body moisturiser or hand cream on yourself
- When making yourself a cup of tea
- When going to your crying baby in the night (bring compassion to you first and then to your baby)
- When wanting to experiment with the power of the compassionate mind by comparing how you might do these things when you are in your compassionate self versus your anxious or irritated self

Your reflections and notes on this section about the qualities of a compassionate mind and the compassionate self practice.

What do you want to hold onto and remember? What would you like to take forward?

____

____

____

____

____

Module 19: Developing our compassionate other/image

Another very powerful way of stimulating our compassion system, this time of imagining receiving compassion, is to create an image of an ideal compassionate being. Because we are creating them in our imagination, they don't need to make any logical sense, so they could be a tree figure, or part-animal/part-human, they could be a combination of somebody we know in real life mixed with a being from a book or a film. We are just constructing the sense of a being that has a mind, with great wisdom, strength and courage who is here just to be with and help us.

As with all these practices, we can have our fears, blocks and resistances that may have developed through our experiences, the way our minds are set up, our particular biology and so on. But being able to receive compassion from others is ultimately exceedingly important for our wellbeing. So even if you may want to skip this, give it a go with a light touch. Let it wash over you and through you as if taking half notice of a song playing in the background. And do keep coming back to it too. It will feel different every time you try it.

Practice: Compassionate other/compassionate image

- Sit with your bottom back in your chair so you feel fully supported, feet flat on the floor, hip width apart (see how bare feet feels). Roll your feet a little until you feel full contact with the floor.
- Sit upright in your 'dignified' posture ('body like a mountain') and gently close your eyes or settle your gaze on an object.
- Imagine warmth or energy bubbling up through the soles of your feet, up your legs, up your spine. Imagine unfurling your spine like a fern in the spring, bringing your shoulders up to your ears, and dropping them back and down, experiencing an openness and spaciousness in your body.

- Now focus on your breath, bringing a warm, kind face, and warm, kind voice to your breath. Perhaps in your mind saying, 'Hello breath!', as if you are really pleased to be with it.
- Slow down your in breath, notice the pause and then really slow down your out breath. In your mind it can help to say slowly on your next out breath, 'breath, slowing, down'. And on your next out breath, saying slowly, 'body, slowing, down'.
- Just notice the feel of this gentle rhythm of breathing in your body, your own soothing breathing rhythm.
- Now imagine that in the distance you become aware of a being or presence that has a feeling of kindness and wisdom about them, and a great strength of character and of courage as if they can stand steady no matter what happens. They have arrived just for you; to help you and support you.
- They might appear as a light, or a colour, or a mist, or as a more distinct image such as a person, an animal or a tree for example. However they appear, they have a mind which is full of kindness, warmth and compassion for you. You may or may not have a clear image of them. This doesn't matter. Just focus on how it feels to have this presence here with you.
- If the image does become clearer you might notice the shape they become, the colour of them, whether they have a face or body. How big or small they are in relation to you.
- Notice what gives you a sense of their kindness.
- You become aware of a sense of their great wisdom, as if they have been around for many years, perhaps hundreds or thousands of years. They have been through many difficult things and are bringing their wisdom here for you.
- You have a sense of their great strength, as if they can withstand anything that life throws at them. They are steady and stable.
- They know you inside and out; there is nothing you need to reveal or disclose to them. They know you and understand you. They understand just how come you are the way you are, including why you might struggle in the particular way you do. They understand too how humans struggle, how we don't choose our genes, or our upbringing, our emotions, our wish to avoid harm and to be safe.

- Notice how they are with you, whether they stay in the distance, sit with you, walk beside you, hold you, whatever it is you need in this moment. If you struggle with their presence, they understand just why this is and they are here to help you and support you in the best way for you.
- If they speak, you might notice the warmth and kindness in their voice. You hear what they say. You notice the expression on their face.
- They may wish to give you something. Notice what it is. A material object? If so, notice how it feels to have it and be given it.
- Notice how it feels to have this kind, warm, strong, wise presence, here just for you. Let the feeling seep into your body.
- Stay with them here as long as you wish.
- You might wish to remember this compassionate being in some way – perhaps giving them a name, or noticing a particular part of them that helps you to recall them.
- Taking this memory in, now shift your attention to the sense of yourself back in your room. Allow the sounds inside and outside your room to enter your ears. Feel the chair solid underneath you. Feel your feet in contact with the ground, begin to move them and feel the floor. Feel your hands, moving them. When you are ready, gently open your eyes.

End of practice.

Reflection:

What was this practice like for you?

___

___

___

What did you find helpful?

Were there any blocks or tricky bits for you?

What might help you with these?

If that fear, block, resistance or tricky bit could be placed on a chair, what might it tell you about its fears? When did the fear first arise? What might its fear be for you if it were to disappear and leave you, or if it went on holiday or went off for a cup of tea when you needed it? How might your compassionate self or compassionate other help it with this fear?

When you might use your compassionate image/other

- When you are struggling to make a decision – you can bring in your compassionate image to support you in your struggle and perhaps bring their wisdom to it.
- When you are going to do something difficult – you might imagine them walking behind you, or next to you, their presence giving you courage. They might say words of encouragement. You know that if it doesn't go as well as you hoped, they would be there to pick you up, understand just how disappointing that is, then help you with it again once you are ready. (One mother was terrified of driving with her new baby in the car. She eventually managed to drive by imagining that her compassionate figure was sitting right behind her.)
- When you are exhausted and would like to have the permission and experience of feeling a little looked after in this moment.
- To sit with you when you are finding it hard to feed your baby.
- To share in your joy.
- To experience their pride in you parenting your baby even when it's hard.

Times when I think my compassionate image/other might help me:

____

____

____

____

____

Troubleshooting the compassionate image/other exercise

This isn't a real person so what is the point?	The power of our imagination is such that we can stimulate the same feeling with a compassionate image as actually being with a compassionate being. Just using imagery can help us to feel safe, loved, give us courage, help us to think differently. It can be very powerful and effective. It then lays down new memories which we can draw on in future. It can also help us to do and think in ways that we struggled with before we did the imagery.
I couldn't get a clear image.	Sometimes people can't bring any image at all. Even just a sense of how it might be and feel if you could be in the presence of this being works.
I couldn't settle on an image.	It can take a number of practices before you begin to find an image that works for you. Once you start thinking about this, you might find you notice people or images in films, on TV, in books or even people you come across in the street. They can all be used to help build your ideal image. You might also need different images at different times.
Can I use a real person?	Real people can prove a little trickier as there may be something about them you wished was a little different. A good test is to think about whether there is anything you wouldn't really want them to know about you. (One mum had her grandmother as her image until she realised that her grandmother wouldn't approve of her swearing!) With imagery you can take bits of real people and merge them with anything you like, take bits out, add bits in, tune bits up or down, to create just the right image for you.
My image keeps changing.	This is usual. In fact, your image may change according to what you need in that moment. One mum wanted to feel small and held and

	cared for; she imagined sitting leaning into the fur of her enormous lion image. But then another time she needed to feel big, strong and confident. This time she imagined a grandfather-type figure based on a kind, wise neighbour who had been high up in the military. He got her to stand up straight, to smooth and straighten her clothes, and marched with her into the situation saying words of encouragement in her ear.
I feel overwhelmingly sad as I never actually had anyone like my image.	Sadness is common and shows just how powerful this is. If you never had anyone in your life like this, then that is terribly sad and it's no wonder you feel this way. Often people go through some grief around this, and you might need some good support while you do. You might want to try different images that don't evoke such sadness. You can also use your compassionate image to help you with your sadness. How would they be with you? How would they support you. How would they help you through this sadness? You can also step into your compassionate image and embody or become them then imagine being with and comforting that sad part of yourself. You have then swapped patterns in your mind and body, from sadness to compassion, so you are no longer fully immersed in the sadness, but you are still addressing it.
I don't believe anyone could really feel compassion or care for me.	You may have never experienced compassion, and this is very sad. It is no wonder you might struggle to believe this compassionate image wants to care for you. This is a very common block for people and is indeed why this whole approach of compassion-focused therapy was developed. The image you develop understands your fears, blocks and resistances and arrives to help you with them. It understands that you

	never chose to feel this way, and that if you had been brought up with different experiences, perhaps in a different family, you may well not feel this way at all – this is not your fault. But it also knows how important it is that you can believe and take in the compassion offered by others, particularly when you have had a baby, so it won't give up and it will continue to stay with you, helping you with this, tiny step by tiny step.
I don't trust them and feel that even if they seem compassionate, they will end up hurting me or letting me down.	Again, this is a common belief and is very sad if this reflects your experiences. This can happen if people you had good relationships with then let you down or had just tried to win you over with fake kindness to be able to take advantage of you. This means that anger, hurt, betrayal, fear and so on, get linked to kindness and compassion so it's no wonder these exercises can get tricky. You may wish to try different compassionate images such as animals, trees, something spiritual like an angel, or Buddha, the sky or the sea, even a car if you feel safe there. It just needs to have a mind that has wisdom, strength and a deep wish to help you as best it can. You may wish to start with 'compassionate self' as this is you being compassionate to yourself and others rather than having to receive it from others. Don't give up on 'compassionate other' though – this may well be your most important practice. This may take time for you to be able to trust your compassionate image, so take it slowly, step by step. Just get used to being in its company. Don't forget it knows you inside and out, and knows just why you struggle to trust it, but it is here just for you, to help you in any way it can. It will never get bored or fed up or frustrated or give up on you. It is here with you whenever you need it.

Your reflections and notes on this section about the compassionate other practice.

What do you want to hold onto and remember? What would you like to take forward?

____

____

____

____

____

Module 20: When it's hard to do compassionate imagery: The power of pretending and acting 'as if'

As humans we can become very constrained by our beliefs about ourselves, particularly if we have grown up with stories that tell us who we are – 'She was always the dramatic one', 'He was always the kindest and most generous of the kids', 'He's the anxious one. His sister has all the guts and courage. She's not scared of anything.' We can also tell ourselves these stories. When we are doing compassionate mind exercises, we can get caught in beliefs that block us here too – 'Yes, but I'm not very strong', 'My sister is the compassionate one. I always preferred to hide my sweets and not share them', 'I'm not at all wise.'

A way of unhooking ourselves from our beliefs is to pretend, to step into the role of somebody who we believe is different from ourselves. We are able to do this because as humans we have this incredible 'new' brain with its ability to imagine. (And even if we are now saying 'Ah, but I don't have a very good imagination', we can pretend; what might it be like if I pretended that I did? Professor of psychology Ellen Langer has made it her life's work to explore this. She calls it the 'power of possibility'. She has created an enormous bank of research around this. A famous piece of research has demonstrated how we can even improve many aspects of our cognitive and physical health by acting as if we are younger than we actually are – see her 'counterclockwise' research.)

Our children enjoy 'putting on' different characters and playing around as them, seeing what they feel like. They can switch really quickly between different ones, and we see how they suddenly start moving differently, using different words, sounding different, having different expressions on their face. As adults we might still do this to a lesser extent when we go into different scenarios, for example acting in an assertive manner when taking something back to a shop even if we don't feel like it inside.

We can even decide we are going to try out a quite different persona when we move into a new environment where we can start afresh with a new story about ourselves, perhaps when we move schools, move house, or when going to college or university.

We can therefore use these principles here with compassionate mind work.

Exercise: Method acting 'as if'

1. Close your eyes or rest your gaze gently on an object, and then bring to mind a part of you that is slightly struggling at the moment. Nothing too much, perhaps a part of you that feels a little tired or headachy or slightly bothered about something. Perhaps something that has been running along in the background while you try to get on with other things. Just allow it to take centre stage for a moment. Allow yourself to see it more clearly and fully. Now imagine that you sit this part next to you. We will call this your 'slightly struggling part'. We will just leave this part here next to us for a moment.
2. Open your eyes and come back into the room.
3. Now write a list of anxious characters from children's television programmes, from films, television series, books, cartoons. Just allow them to pop into your mind.

____

____

____

____

____

4. Now make a list of compassionate characters from children's television programmes, from films, television programmes, cartoons, books. Just see who pops into your mind.

____

____

____

____

____

5. Now pick one of the anxious characters. Imagine that you are a method actor who has been studying this character for months. You have been studying how this character moves, the clothes they wear (if they wear clothes), how they sound if they speak, how they interact with others, how others react to them. Now imagine bending down and stepping your feet into their feet and pulling up their body and clothes as if you are literally stepping into their body. Then simply move around the room as this anxious character. Let yourself do this for a few minutes. Note what this is like as you are doing it.
6. Now come up to your 'slightly struggling part' seated in the chair, and just relate to it as your anxious character. Spend a few minutes with it.

Your reflections on this:

What was this like as you moved around the room as your anxious character?

____

____

____

____

How did you feel in yourself?

____

____

____

____

How were you moving?

____

____

____

____

What thoughts were coming into your mind?

What did you pay attention to?

What did you notice when you came to your slightly struggling part?

How did you feel towards it?

What was your urge in your body?

____

____

____

____

If this urge were to grow and grow, what would your anxious character really want to do if it could?

____

____

____

____

What did your anxious character want to say to the slightly struggling part?

____

____

____

____

7. Now take off your anxious character, stepping out of it as if you are stepping out of dressing-up clothes. Pick one of the compassionate characters from your list. Again, as a method actor, you have been studying this character for months, observing how it moves, how it walks, the clothes it wears if it wears any, how it sounds if it speaks, how it relates to others and how they relate to it. Imagine bending down and stepping your feet into its feet, and pulling up its body and clothes so you are now standing in its body. Now just walk and move around the room as this character. Take your time noticing how it feels to be this character. Spend a few minutes moving about the room.
8. Now just approach the slightly struggling part of yourself. Nothing to do here but just relate to it from your compassionate character. Spend a few minutes here with your slightly struggling self.

Your reflections on this:

What was this like as you moved around the room as your compassionate character?

How did you feel in yourself?

How were you moving?

What thoughts were coming into your mind?

What did you pay attention to?

What did you notice when you came to your slightly struggling part?

How did you feel towards it?

What was your urge in your body?

If this urge were to grow and grow, what would your compassionate character really want to do if it could?

What did your compassionate character want to say to the slightly struggling part?

What do you imagine your slightly struggling part would have experienced when your *anxious* character spent time with it?

What do you imagine your slightly struggling part would have experienced when your *compassionate* character spent time with it?

Now take off your compassionate character, stepping out of it as if you are stepping out of dressing-up clothes (or keep it on if you wish!).

Your overall reflections on this exercise. What would you like to take hold of and remember from this?

Your reflections and notes on this section about method acting and the power of acting 'as if'.

What do you want to hold onto and remember? What would you like to take forward?

Module 21: Compassionate desensitisation – bringing compassion to our 'ladder' of compassionate mind practices

People usually have favourite compassionate mind practices, easy practices, practices they find hard and practices they discard. Often the most difficult ones turn out to be the ones we need the most. You are likely to have an intuitive sense of how you might help your baby with something they are scared of or find difficult. We can bring this process to ourselves too.

How might you help your baby if they had been barked at by a big dog and were now really scared of going out of the house?

____

____

____

____

In this example, you might first make sure that there are no dogs outside the house, and just open the front door and sit with your baby on your lap, showing them that it's safe. Once they are calmer you then might carry them down the path, talking gently and encouragingly to them. You are intuitively using your body, voice tone and facial expression to bring online their soothing safeness system. This feeling of safeness is then being connected to going outside and overlays the threat feelings. These feelings of safeness whilst being outside become new memories.

You then might take them out in their buggy rather than holding them. Talking to them. Pointing out things that interest them – showing them that it is a world that they want to be in.

As their safeness and confidence builds you might start to take them to places where they can see dogs in the far distance, again talking with your warm, kind face and voice, explaining, encouraging, bringing the feelings of safeness and courage to your child.

You then might, over time, bring them closer to dogs, perhaps arranging for a friend's gentle dog to come over and play in the garden while you hold your baby. Working all the way up this 'ladder' of difficulty for your child, so that in the end they are able to do what is important for them to be able to live well in the world. This is helping them to live fully in their lives, even if some residual anxiety around particular dogs remains.

Doing this for your child is a truly compassionate act. Without it they could (and many of us do) live their entire lives in a scared and restricted way, eventually with unimaginable levels of impact upon almost every aspect of their lives.

We can apply exactly the same process to our own fears, no matter what age, or how entrenched these fears are. Here we are looking at applying it specifically to tricky aspects of these practices and of compassionate mind work.

Just like we would do with our baby or child if they are trying to master something;

- Start with something that isn't too hard and isn't too easy. So, we are pushing ourselves in order to create new learning, but not so much that we become overwhelmed or give up.
- We are working up the 'ladder' of difficulty. This will be the first 'rung'. We can make the distance between each rung just about right for ourselves. Our compassionate mind can help us to bring the creativity we might need to this process. We can use our imagination, drawings, photos, toys, the internet, real life, recruit the help of others in order to help us face each step of our fear.
- As well as engaging with each rung of the fear, we also need to bring a body experience of safeness, support, soothing and compassion to it. We are creating a new association of safeness instead of fear, so we need to be able to feel this safeness, which then creates new memories.
- Experiment with bringing your compassionate self to this and then try bringing your compassionate image or other to this. You might switch between both.
- Try it without your compassionate mind with you and see how it compares. Does the compassionate mind make a difference?

- The compassion aspect is important; after all, we are doing something that we find hard and probably scary or anxiety provoking so it will take a great deal of the strength and courage aspect of our compassionate mind. Our compassionate mind provides us with the 'secure base' that allows us to move out and engage with what we fear.
- We also need to bring the understanding, support and kindness aspect of our compassionate mind to ourselves, particularly if we don't manage what we hoped. As well as a 'secure base', our compassionate mind provides a 'safe haven' where we have an understanding, supportive, soothing and settling mind which helps us with our disappointment and helps to calm and regulate our upset.
- This helps our mind and body come back to a state where we can try again. The wisdom of the compassionate mind helps us to understand what might have happened this time, and how to tweak and change it for next time.
- The strength of our compassionate mind helps to ensure that we don't give up, as it knows in the long run just how important this will be for us, and perhaps even for our baby and others too. Instead, it stands by us, getting ready to support and encourage us with it another time.
- Our compassionate mind can help us with our compassion motivation for what we are trying to do. It helps us to become clearer and clearer about just why we want this for ourselves, and specifically what will look and feel different to ourselves and others as we overcome each fear. The clarity helps us keep our mind focused on those distant goals like a flag we set on a distant mountain – that's where we are taking ourselves. Each step towards it will bring something new, to ourselves, our baby, and those around us.

So, we might want to come back to the trickier practices again and again, especially as we work through this book. As we do, we bring our kindness and compassion to ourselves especially if it's difficult – it will be difficult for a good reason, but it will be worth the benefit as we master them.

Imagine trying something difficult *without* your compassionate mind with you (e.g. going with your baby on your own to a parent and baby group – anything you would like to do but find challenging).

How might you set about trying to do this difficult thing?

What would keep you going if you were finding it hard?

Without a compassionate mind, what would you be like towards yourself if you succeeded?

Without a compassionate mind, what would you be like towards yourself if you didn't succeed?

Now imagine having your compassionate self/compassionate image/compassionate mind with you.

How might you set about trying to do this difficult thing? How might your compassionate mind help you?

____

____

____

____

What would keep you going if you were finding it hard? How might your compassionate mind be with you?

____

____

____

____

What would it be like if you succeeded? How might your compassionate mind be with you?

____

____

____

____

How would it be if you didn't succeed? How might your compassionate mind be with you?

Reflections and notes: What would you like to take hold of and remember from this section about compassionate systematic desensitisation and how we might use it to help us with things we might fear, including particular compassionate mind practices? What would you like to take forward and try? What might be your next steps?

Section 4:

The impact on the brain of becoming a mother

Module 22: Brain changes during pregnancy

When we become pregnant, the changes that occur within our body are phenomenal. Such a lot of a woman's body exists for this time of creating, growing and raising an entirely new human being. The intricacies and complexities of this have been finely honed over millions of years of evolution. After all, reproduction is the most important aspect of all for the future of our species.

Although some of the physical changes are obvious, it is not until relatively recently that we have started to become aware of the changes that occur within the brain of a pregnant woman too. Brain scans have shown that, compared to a non-pregnant woman's brain scanned over the same period, a pregnant woman's brain appears to shrink in size. The changes are in the grey matter made of neurons – the 'wiring' of the brain. Rather than brain loss however, this indicates that the brain is becoming highly specialised. In other words, the parts of the brain that are going to be particularly needed for growing and bringing up a baby become more developed and more efficiently connected. The change is so dramatic that it is easy to look at brain scans and pick the brain that has experienced pregnancy from the brain that hasn't.

Changes on a scan don't however tell us what this actually means for the woman that is, or has been, pregnant. The researchers therefore compared the degree of change on the scan over the course of pregnancy with the degree of how positively the woman described her baby and how she interacted with her baby. The greater the changes in the grey matter of the brain, the more positively the woman described her baby, the more sensitive and attuned were her interactions with her baby, and the more securely attached the baby became. The areas of the brain that changed were those that have repeatedly been found to be associated with different aspects of parenting, such as a motivation to parent, understanding the mind of others as separate to our own, sensitivity of interaction, and attuned interactions.

Changes that have been noticed previously across pregnancy include an increased awareness of emotions felt by others as pregnancy progresses and an increased interest in and understanding of the minds of others. This accumulation of evidence suggests that the changes within the pregnant body are also preparing the brain to meet, want to interact with, want to care for, and want to understand the new baby. It is quite incredible. All without us choosing for this to happen, and in fact whether we like it or not.

Although these changes are highly selected through evolution, it doesn't necessarily mean we experience it as all good. It may be, for example, that we are already very sensitive to emotions in others, and that this increase through pregnancy feels overwhelming.

The changes are so marked that some have likened it to the degree of change that occurs after a serious brain injury. However, for somebody who has had such a brain injury, it is accepted that we have to learn how our brain now works. We may have to re-learn and re-train ourselves. We understand that the process of rapid change can cause fatigue, and requires much rest to allow new learning to become embedded and crystallised by the brain – much like a baby requiring a great deal of sleep and zoning out in order to have time to lay down this new learning in their brain. However, in motherhood, this process of becoming a mother, including developing this new brain, is rarely held in awe, or given time, space, rest or support. And of course, these enormous brain changes are taking place whilst a woman is also learning how to take care of a completely dependent baby. Whilst we wait for our society to hopefully catch up with this understanding, we can at least set about regarding ourselves with awe, compassion and acceptance, and give ourselves time to work out what we need and how to get it as best we can.

What I need to help my brain and body to adjust to having a new baby:

____

____

____

____

For example:

- Some mental 'down-time' like my baby has – some time just to stare out of the window and watch the birds or the clouds or go for a walk whilst someone looks after my baby.
- Some time to just chat about the changes to friends or family.

- Working out a rhythm with my partner or family so I get some more sleep.
- Napping while my baby sleeps during the day.
- Arranging to have fewer visitors.
- Arranging to have more visitors.
- When people ask 'just let me know how I can help', having a list ready (people really do want to help – it can be an evolved need, as a new baby would have been highly valuable to the small groups we used to live in for much of our human existence): e.g. to cook us some meals, to hold the baby for an hour so I can do some of the cooking, baking, crafts, gardening, cleaning, reading, walking, running, that I would like to do, to write out a meal plan for us, to sort out the house insurance / gas reading / other admin that I just can't get to do at the moment, to pick my other child up from school / take them to school once a week, to mow the lawn so we can go in the garden . . .

Reflections and notes: What would you like to take hold of and remember from this section about brain changes during pregnancy? What would you like to take forward and try? What might be your next steps?

____

____

____

____

Module 23: Brain changes after pregnancy

Rapid brain changes also occur after pregnancy. Instead of the brain appearing to shrink on brain scans as it seems to during pregnancy, following pregnancy it appears to grow. This is thought to be due to the enormous number of new experiences and learning that occurs in caring for, interacting with, and trying to work out how to best parent this new baby. The brain has an incredibly 'plastic' nature where it responds to the environment it is operating within (called 'neuroplasticity'). It continues changing throughout our lives. This means that even if the mother's brain has not had the same degree of change as another mother's brain during pregnancy, just the experience of looking after a baby will be creating vast and rapid changes in the brain anyway. It just might feel a little harder and take more conscious effort (or it might not – we just don't know enough about these changes yet).

So, all of what we will be covering here is about consciously creating a brain and body that supports us to flourish, supports us in parenting, and supports us in helping our baby to flourish too. Even if, and especially if, for whatever reason we don't have quite the brain changes, or the upbringing, or anything else that might make motherhood a little easier.

Such changes also occur in the brain of whoever else is closely involved in caring for the baby, such as dad, partner, grandparent, adoptive parents, foster parents, neonatal nurses. Interestingly, these changes in grandmothers seemed to relate to how much they *want* to be involved with their grandchild, regardless of how much they are actually able to be involved. It seems, therefore, that the wish or motivation is important, not just the actual experiences we are having. So back again to the compassion motivation.

This motivational system is so important. It really is the place that we move off from, even if there are not the feelings that usually accompany and assist it. Very often mothers are trying to do the very best for their baby even if they don't feel very much for them, are depressed, or even feel dislike towards them. It is quite astonishing – this requires such compassion to be still striving to connect, love, care for and bond with our baby when there isn't so much of the biology such as feelings of warmth, love, oxytocin flow or maternal urge to parent, that makes it so much easier.

This wish, intention, motivation, drive to find a way to make the relationship with the baby better is the key.

The feelings will follow on.

These brain changes occur along with hormonal changes, regardless of gender. Typically, the involved partner experiences a lowering in testosterone and raising of oxytocin, reflecting and fostering an increasing bond with the baby.

Reflections: What would you like to take hold of and remember from this part?

____

____

____

____

Alloparenting: Sharing the care of our baby

That physiological changes occur in all those caring for the baby is particularly important in humans, where we appear to be relatively unusual within primates in that we (and a handful of other primates) share the care of our offspring. It is thought to be a key reason why we have become such a successful species – because if we are looked after as mothers, and have help with our children, we are much more able to raise our offspring to the age when they can reproduce. We can also have babies in quick succession. Mammals that don't have help and are the sole carers have to wait a substantial number of years between offspring, until their existing offspring are independent of them. Whereas human mothers, with additional help, can have another baby when her other child is still a baby or a young, still dependent, child. This means that humans can reproduce quickly, a very important evolutionary strategy.

But to share the care, we need to be within a network that is interested in and invested in us and our baby – this was much easier when we lived in small tribes, or villages where our relations and friends were close by, and where a new baby was seen as a highly valuable addition to the pool of genes and to the size of that small group. This was especially important when lives were short and dangers due to famine, other animals, disease and so on were high. It is much harder to share the care of the baby now in societies where it is difficult to even see and spend time with a new mother and her baby, let alone help with the care. For our families to be able to flourish according to their evolutionary wiring, we need communities that fit with this wiring. If we cannot have this, then at least we can bring compassion to ourselves, that it is not our fault that we struggle when we don't have additional help. 'Additional help' for most of our human existence may have been as many as ten core carers for a baby, so we also need compassion to ourselves when we and our partner are not managing – even the two of you working together well is not enough. This really is not your fault.

Your reflections on 'sharing the care of your baby'.

____

____

____

____

A note on the difference between guilt and shame

When we have a baby, it seems that they arrive with a special 'parcel' of guilt too. It might seem that we have never experienced such levels and frequency of guilt until we have a baby. We might feel guilty that we've not eaten the right foods during pregnancy, that we aren't quick enough to respond to our baby's cries, that we have secret wishes to be free to do what we did before our baby came, that we want to give up breastfeeding, that we are going back to work when we feel we should stay at home, or that we have given up work when really we need the money . . .

Well, there is a very good reason why guilt and our baby seem so entwined. This is because they are both linked to the same system: the soothing/safeness system which is underpinned by the motivation for care-giving and care-receiving. Guilt arises when we feel that we have not been as helpful as we could, or that we have been unintentionally harmful. We feel bad about our behaviour or our thoughts *because we care*. If we go back to Paul Gilbert's definition of compassion, 'To be helpful, not harmful', we need a system that enables us to check whether, even when we intended to be helpful, we actually were. So, for example, we might pick up a toy when our baby was trying to master reaching for it for themselves and they get frustrated with us. We need a mechanism that allows us to see the response in the other person to our behaviour but also to be moved to do something about it and make it right. The feeling of guilt alerts us to the fact that our baby wasn't happy with what we did, and we might then apologise and repair it. We might say, '*Oh you wanted to do that yourself. I am sorry*', then perhaps help them once again to reach and get the toy themselves. Perhaps we get annoyed with our baby when they are in their deliberately dropping everything over the edge of the highchair stage, and talk to them sharply. Again, the horrible feeling that we call 'guilt' brings our attention to this and drives us to want to make it better. We might say, '*I am sorry. I know this isn't your fault and I am sorry I was sharp with you. You can do three more "drops" but then that will do for now. I'll get you out and put you on the floor so you can drop and pick things up as many times as you want to.*'

With our new brain ability to imagine, we can also play out in our mind how our behaviour might affect another person, even if we hadn't actually behaved that way in real life. We can therefore feel guilty even about our thoughts, images or urges. But we can also make use of our imagination by changing our behaviour to try to make it better and then replay in our imagination how this new behaviour might turn out. This is in fact the basis of what we will be talking about later in terms of the 'dance' with our baby. We are all the time monitoring and adjusting our interactions with our baby, as are they with us. This responsivity in us creates the basis of a secure attachment (as well as many other incredible benefits).

Your examples of guilt (they don't need to be yours, just examples to help understand this)**.**

____

____

____

____

Shame, on the other hand, is very different to guilt. When you feel ashamed, notice what happens in your body. It can make us feel anxious, collapsed, like we want the ground to 'swallow us up'. We are worried about people finding out about what we are ashamed about and, if they did find out, we fear being cast out. Our urge is to hide shameful feelings, to tuck them away deep inside. We are now very firmly in our threat system when shame hits. Unlike with guilt, our urge is not to reach out, reconnect, say sorry, make amends. Rather, it is to retreat, to hide, to pull away. Whereas guilt is usually about a specific thought, feeling or behaviour – 'I did this wrong, and I feel bad about it. I am sorry' – shame sweeps through us and feels like it is about our very self – 'I *am* bad'.

In the example of giving the toy when our baby wanted to reach it themselves, a shame response might be, 'I always get this wrong. I am so useless at this. And now he hates me.' Our urge might be to distance ourselves from our baby and to make sure that nobody sees us trying to play with them. In the example of speaking crossly to our baby when they drop their toys repeatedly, shame might drive us to think, 'Oh my goodness, I can't believe I got cross with them for doing what babies do. I am just rubbish at this and a horrible person.' Again, the urge might be to withdraw and spend less time with our baby, and to use our critic to make sure we never get angry with our baby again. Shame is such a horrible and harmful experience.

Your examples of shame (they don't need to be yours, again, just examples to help understand this).

____

____

____

____

The aim is to be able to move from shame to guilt, because then we can reach out and repair and mend the relationship again. This is where we need our compassionate mind. Our compassionate mind de-shames us by helping us to understand that our thoughts, behaviours, urges and so on are just part of the human condition. These are not our fault and make complete sense given the brain and body given to us by evolution and by the experiences and genes that have shaped us but that we didn't choose. As we realise we are part of this human species, part of the world and part of the line of mothers extending backwards into the past, forwards into the future, and all around the world, trying to manage as best they can, we can feel connected again. With connection comes safeness. With safeness comes the brain shift that enables us to hold in mind our baby and bring compassion to ourselves and then compassion to our baby. Without the shame we can experience the guilt, and the corresponding urge to reach out to them again, reconnect, make amends and carry on the to and fro of interactions, from a place of best intentions.

We will be looking at ways to work with shame throughout the book.

Your reflections on guilt and shame: What do you want to hold onto and remember from this?

What if I struggle to like or connect with my baby?

The question on many mothers' minds may now be, but what if my brain hasn't changed? What does it mean if I don't feel attuned to my baby, or don't feel love or don't even feel that I like my baby? What if I feel like my baby isn't mine, as if I've been given the wrong baby at birth? These experiences are so hard and so sad. And babies require such a great deal of care and thought, that how do we manage this when, for whatever reason (and there are many reasons including chronic stress, a lack of support, depression, trauma, a difficult and exhausting birth, difficult early life experiences, neurodiversity and so on), the brain set-up, the hormones and so on that help and support this, haven't happened for us? It really can seem like some kind of miracle that women relentlessly struggle on doing the best they can. Sometimes this is at great cost to both the physical and mental health of the mother.

The studies show the degree of variance in women's brains over pregnancy, so this of course invites the question about what influences the degree of change. This research is still so new that it isn't really well known. However, studies are finding that chronic stress, depression, anxiety, lack of sleep, lack of support, and trauma can influence maternal brain changes.

In addition, it may be that the brain changes in themselves may put women more at risk of developing mood and anxiety disorders. So, for example, it seems like the brains of mothers change to become more flexible and adaptable generally, perhaps to be able to respond quickly to changes in situations particularly regarding their baby. The changes also occur in areas which give rise to increased vigilance, protectiveness, threat detection and preoccupation with the infant. This allows for adaptive checking and worrying behaviours, for example. However, these brain networks overlap with those involved in anxiety, fear and mood disorders, suggesting that maternal brain changes may mean mothers are more at risk of developing these.

There are also quite phenomenal hormonal changes that occur during pregnancy and that then plummet rapidly after pregnancy, or flux during breastfeeding or when breastfeeding is stopped. These can all impact upon mood, again creating increased potential for mood disorders.

And on top of all this, there is a hypothesis that being pregnant itself creates a natural inflammatory response and that this is greater when pregnant with a boy than a girl. A painful and traumatic birth or painful breastfeeding may cause more inflammation. There is now growing evidence that some depression is linked to inflammation in the body.

This is all without considering the impact of the pregnancy and the birth, levels of exhaustion, feeling physically unwell, amount of support the mother has, and the baby itself. In addition to any background factors such as attachment history, previous mental health difficulties, circumstances around conception such as IVF and so on and so on. So many factors will influence a mother's relationship with her baby, and how she feels about her baby.

What is so tragic is that often mothers blame themselves for being depressed or anxious or stressed. As we can see, this is not their fault. Instead of blame and shame, the way out is through compassion, support and professional help if necessary.

The vast majority of mothers have no mood or anxiety disorders though, and indeed for many having a baby is a positive experience, and can even buffer against anxiety and depression.

As we can see, this is just a tiny insight into just how complex this perinatal time is for mothers. What is clear though is that safeness is imperative. This is why the compassionate mind approach has been taken up in so many perinatal services – because regardless of causes, the biological and brain impact of safeness has a profoundly significant impact on mothers, and their connections and interactions with their baby.

This is also why so much attention, and money, is at long last being focused on women's mental and physical health, particularly during pregnancy and the postpartum period. It is such a tragedy for mothers to suffer in this way at such an important time. And often a little extra support, information or guidance is all that is needed to give mothers, as well as their partners, the best start possible in the process of parenthood. So, if this is a concern to you, do contact your midwife, health visitor or GP to discuss the help available to you.

This area will also be addressed in more detail later in the book.

Your reflections on this section: What do you want to hold onto and remember from this?

____

____

____

____

'Golden window'– Perinatal as a time of particular brain neuroplasticity

The perinatal period is sometimes referred to as a 'golden window' of opportunity as there seems to be something about this time in a woman's life when she is particularly susceptible to the impact of interventions and change. It may be the brain changes, hormonal changes, the motivation of doing it for the baby, the openness that is created by having another being inside of us. Whatever it is, it is well known that sometimes just a little bit of help at this time can create much greater changes than at other times in our life. Perhaps it needs more than a little help. But this really is a good time to seek help. And the earlier the better. But if it is no longer 'earlier', then still pursue help. Things can change profoundly at any point in our life. And we know from neuroplasticity research that we can change and shape our brain throughout our life. Indeed, the exercises that we will be doing in this book are brain changing – which is why they are referred to as 'compassionate mind training'. The more you do them, the greater the change, and the more likely you will be able to respond with greater calm and steadiness.

We also need to know how best to buffer against stress, depression, anxiety and trauma during pregnancy and the postnatal period, and what will best help us if sadly we do experience these things on top of being pregnant and looking after a new baby. Sleep is also vitally important in terms of brain functioning with regard to our baby (see later in the book for ways to help sleep), on top of many other crucial aspects. This book aims to offer some powerful ways of helping with these as well as helping families to access additional support during this significant time. Compassion isn't just about how we are with ourselves, but is also about allowing ourselves to access and take in the compassion and help offered by others.

When women are experiencing these difficulties, they can feel shame and self-criticism. Especially when so often on TV and in social media we see new mothers 'snapping back' to pre-baby weight, doing wonderful activities with their baby, apparently always adoring their baby and loving motherhood. This can add to the sense of shame and increase self-criticism, particularly as this is a time when we actually need more help and social contact. This can result in loneliness and also an anxiety of being on the margins, ready to be 'cast out' any minute if people were to discover how we really felt about our baby and being a mother. We already know that being cast out is an ancient, evolved terror for humans as for most of our life as humans we wouldn't have survived if we were. But we also know that human mothers have evolved to share the care of their baby. So, this terror may be even greater for new mothers where being part of the group is even more important.

However, if we stay in shame and self-criticism then we become too scared to connect with others for fear of what they might discover, leaving us trapped in aloneness. Instead, what would it be like to swap systems from a threat mind to our compassionate mind?

Professor Paul Gilbert has developed the compassionate mind approach and compassion-focused therapy specifically as a way of helping us when we experience high shame, self-criticism and its resulting anxiety and depression.

Revisit the practice of either compassionate self or compassionate other at this point. These take practice, sometimes a great deal, so let whichever one you choose just play through you loosely and gently at first, just noticing with interest and warmth anything that arises in you. If you want, you can imagine it just playing in the background, like quiet music.

Reflections and notes: What would you like to take hold of and remember from this section about brain changes after pregnancy, the difference between guilt and shame, the potential struggle to connect to our baby and the perinatal period as a 'golden window' in terms of neuroplasticity? What would you like to take forward and try? What might be your next steps?

____

____

____

____

____

Module 24: Matrescence – 'I have become a mother'

This change to becoming a mother has been called 'matrescence', to recognise it as a stage in its own right. Like other life stages or transitions such as adolescence, we are understanding more and more the extent of the brain-body changes that occur, the reasons these changes might be occurring, and how best to support this process.

As humans we can find change challenging. We find change easiest when we feel safe and scaffolded enough to move with the change. This means, as ever, moving into the safeness/soothing system which calms our anxiety about change, but also allows us to access the part of our brain which helps us to lay down new learning. It is also the part of the brain that is involved in our sense of our self-identity – so in other words the soothing/safeness system helps us to lay down the sense of 'I have become a mother' in our brain.

Practice: Compassionate brain 'smoothing and soothing'

After all these words and talk of the need to have space for our brain, mind and bodies to adjust to motherhood, here is a quick practice to 'smooth' and sooth the brain.

- Sit with your back straight, feet hip width apart and connected to the floor (try bare feet).
- Close your eyes or settle your gaze gently on an object, keeping your head facing forwards.
- Bring your shoulders up to your ears, drop them back and down, opening your chest.
- Slow your in breath, and really slow down your out breath.
- Bring a warm, kind face and warm, kind voice to your breath, perhaps saying, 'Hello breath'. Notice as it begins to move into its own slow, deep, smooth, soothing rhythm.

- Imagine now, a light, colour, or mist appears. You feel it has arrived just for you.
- It seems to have a warmth, kindness and compassion about it.
- Imagine that it comes in through the top of your head, washing over your brain like a tropical rain shower: warm, soft, gentle.
- Imagine it smoothing down any areas that feel particularly frazzled, tired or irritable, like the smoothing of a sheet on a bed, or the fur on a cat or a dog or furry blanket.
- Connect with a sense of just how it might feel for the brain to be smoothed and soothed in this way; perhaps it is gratitude and relief.
- Enjoy this moment of soothing, of smoothing. Stay with this as long as you wish.
- When you are ready, tune back in to the sounds around you, the feel of whatever you are sitting on supporting you, the feel of your feet in contact with the floor and the feel of your hands – perhaps moving them both.
- When you are ready, gently open your eyes.

End of practice.

Your reflections on this practice: What do you want to hold onto and remember from this?

____

____

____

____

Practice: Compassion to my new mother's body

As we go through pregnancy not only does our brain change, but our body changes in quite astonishing ways. Many of these changes are permanent. Even our feet become permanently bigger. We really do 'become a mother' even if sadly we lose our baby. Like the Japanese concept of kintsugi (where broken pottery is mended with gold to bring attention and appreciation to the beauty and value of the story of the pot, including breakages), our body takes on the story of our physical journey of becoming a mother.

- Sit in a 'dignified' posture with your back and head upright, your feet hip width apart and in contact with the floor. Bring your shoulders up to your ears, then drop them back and down. Feel the openness and increase in space in your body.
- Bring your warm, kind face, and warm, kind voice to your breath, as if you are really pleased to have encountered it. Perhaps in your mind say, 'Hello breath!'. Allow your in breath to deepen and then allow your out breath to pour all the way out, slow and smooth, from the base of your lungs, all the way out into the air. Breathe in again slow and smooth, just enjoying the sensation of allowing your breath to slow down. You might notice that it settles into its own soothing rhythm. As it does you might notice an increase in your sense of stability and steadiness in your body.
- Tune into the part of you that is caring, helpful, compassionate. The part of you that has great wisdom, which has been through many things, has learned so much both formally in education, through training, but also through people you've encountered, books you've read, films and TV programmes you have watched. You deeply understand the difficulties and wonder of having this human brain and body, that you did not choose but that has been shaped by millions of years of evolution, your experiences, your genes, the process of pregnancy. You have great strength and courage, perhaps more than you imagined, meaning you tackle and get through some very difficult things.
- Bring your kind, warm, compassionate mind to your head, perhaps placing your hand gently on your head. Allow your hand to send in warmth and compassion to your brain that has changed so much and to your mind that is working so hard with this new task

of mothering. Imagine how your brain feels to be noticed in this way. Allow it to receive and take in your gratitude and compassion.

- Bring your attention now to your face, your jaw, your lips, your tongue. All working so hard to communicate with your baby. Perhaps bringing your hands to cup your face, feeling your warmth and compassion easing into your face. Sense your face receiving this compassion.
- Now bring your compassionate mind to your chest and your breasts, perhaps placing your hands on or over them. Send compassion to your breasts, your heart, your lungs that have been changing and working so hard. Sense the feeling of them receiving your warmth, your compassion, your gratitude.
- Shift your compassionate mind to your stomach, perhaps laying your hands on or over it. This part that has carried a new life, even if for a short while. This uterus and even the gut bacteria within you, having changed and adapted so much. This skin that has had to stretch so much and may bear marks of this and of the darkening from hormonal changes. These muscles that have had to open, stretch and carry this weight. Bringing your warmth and your compassion to seep in deep to all of these parts. You might take in how these parts feel to be given this compassion, to be noticed in this way.
- Move the attention of your compassionate mind to your arms and to your hands that do so much for you, for your baby, for others. Feel the compassion flow all the way down your arms, into the palms of your hands, into each finger and your thumbs. Allow these parts to receive this warm, compassionate attention.
- Shift your compassionate attention to your bladder, your cervix, your bottom. Perhaps place your hand over or on them. Allow the compassion to ease into these parts that have been impacted so much by carrying and delivering a baby. Sense how these parts might feel to receive this warm, kind, compassionate attention.
- Bring your compassionate attention to your legs, your knees, your ankles, your feet, your toes. These parts of you that carry you, support you, and your baby, that change during pregnancy, becoming wider, adding to your steadiness. Bring your compassionate attention to any changes in your skin, or the veins on your legs. Place your hands on

or over these different parts of your body. Notice how these parts feel to be given this compassion.

- Now expand your attention out to take in your body, brain, and mind as a whole. Bring your compassionate attention to the whole of it, this new body and brain of a mother. A body and brain that becomes part of this group of mothers around the world, back in time through the ages of millions of mothers, and forward in time to all the mothers to come.
- See what it might be like to send compassion out to all these mothers here now in the world, those that have gone, and those to come. You might notice what it might be like for them to be given this compassionate attention.
- Notice what it is like for the mother that is you to be included in this group. Notice how it feels for her (you) to take in this compassionate attention.
- Stay with this for as long as you wish.
- When you are ready, tune in to the sounds around you, inside your room and outside your room. Allow them to gently flow in through your ears. Shift your attention to the feel of the chair holding you up, then the feel of your hands in your lap and your feet on the floor, perhaps wiggling them. When you are ready, gently open your eyes. You may wish to stretch and move about. See if you can take this feeling of compassion in your body to accompany you as best you can as you go about your day.

End of practice.

Your reflections on this practice: What do you want to hold onto and remember from this?

____

____

____

____

Reflections and notes: What would you like to take hold of and remember from this section about matrescense and bringing compassion to the changes to your brain and body? What would you like to take forward and try? What might be your next steps?

____

____

____

____

____

Module 25: Sleep

Sleep deprivation can be a particularly difficult aspect of having a new baby. Although it is seen as a normal part of this stage, it is only 'normal' where there is lack of support. For most of our human history a baby crying at night would have been a magnet for predators, putting not just the baby, but the whole group, at risk. It is likely that, for thousands of years of our human evolution, at night there would be close human contact and the presence of a group highly invested in one another, all sleeping in one space. There may well have been at least one person awake 'on watch' at night for danger. Sleep is a very vulnerable state and the need for somebody watching out for danger on our behalf, particularly when we have a baby, may well be hardwired into us. This sleep set-up would provide the safeness and responsivity that facilitates sleep for both mother and baby.

> Lack of sleep in the perinatal period can increase the risk of postpartum depression and anxiety and is also a risk factor in postpartum psychosis and bipolar disorder. If you find that you are waking in the early hours of the morning, even when your baby is asleep, particularly if you are finding you have anxious, depressed or racing thoughts, then contact your GP or midwife immediately. The quicker you can get treatment if you are developing a psychiatric illness related to childbirth the more likely a potentially more serious episode can be averted. If you are not sure whether or not there is anything to worry about, still see your midwife, health visitor or GP as soon as you can, to talk it over. They are trained to be checking all postnatal women for signs of perinatal mental illness so will be taking you seriously and can get you treatment quickly if needed. They can also keep a closer eye on you to monitor you (sometimes known as 'watchful waiting'), which can often be very helpful in itself.

Even what might be considered a relatively minor loss of sleep after having a baby will be having an impact. Just one night of sleep deprivation or routinely getting six hours of sleep or less is associated with increases in anxiety and depression in healthy individuals. The research is showing that this may be to do with weakening activity in the pre-frontal cortex, along with its connection to the amygdala. The amygdala is the area that mounts a threat response or prepares the body to deal with novelty. The pre-frontal cortex allows us to have a 'top down' control over this (see Dan Siegel's lovely little video on the internet explaining his 'hand model of the brain' and 'flipping our lid'). This means that after relatively little sleep disturbance, the amygdala can create a strong emotional response without the pre-frontal cortex being able to damp it down. Participants in one study who had six hours of sleep or less were found to have equally strong responses when shown bland images of commuters on a train as they were to images of children crying. Well-rested participants only had amygdala responses to the images of children crying. So, for parents who routinely have disrupted sleep, it is no wonder they may feel more emotional, anxious and depressed even with regard to seemingly 'bland' events, let alone about their crying baby.

The pre-frontal cortex is also important in how we mentalise (think about and understand the minds of others) so this can impact how we relate to our babies, to others in our lives, and even to ourselves. Yet sleep deprivation is often regarded as just the lot of parents. Something which you just have to get on and deal with. Almost a badge you must wear. The impact it can have is not taken particularly seriously. Yet once people get enough sleep then all these things affected by sleep are put right again. It can be quite extraordinary to discover just how much of what we had been struggling with was just down to lack of sleep.

We have seen the degree of brain changes that occur in mothers and other involved caregivers to the baby. We know that babies need a great deal of sleep to support the brain changes and the enormous degree of learning that is happening to them each day too. Parents also need sleep for the same reasons. It is not just important for our mental health but for the laying down of new memories and new learning; essential when learning new skills of parenting, and of parenting *this* baby. It is also important to our physical health, including conditions such as diabetes, heart disease, high blood pressure, as well as healing up after birth and the regulation of insulin, which is connected to weight gain.

So given good sleep is a priority for parents, what might help to improve sleep?

Ways to improve our sleep as parents

- Accept offers of help, particularly with regard to enabling sleep.
- Looking after a new baby is demanding, an enormous responsibility, and requires as sharp a mind as possible. Good sleep is therefore required. But often the sleep of the partner who is returning to work is prioritised. Both parents need sleep, so working out how this can happen is crucial. Having people come to stay, having baby looked after once a week at grandparents, parents sleeping in 'shifts', or one going to bed early in the evening to get in a long chunk of sleep before taking over from the other can all be invaluable solutions for this short-term issue (although it may not feel short-term when we are in the midst of it).

- Like our baby, even as adults we need to prepare our body and brain for the transition from awake to asleep. What works for our baby, works for us too – so a clear routine that we do every night that signals sleep time, and 'steps' our brain down and down for sleep. Each step becomes associated with each level of sleepiness. (One mum used to say that no matter how seemingly wide awake her baby was, as soon as she put him in his sleep suit, he'd start yawning. Perhaps similar to us when put on our pyjamas.)
- Sleep is triggered by environmental cues such as temperature and light, so keep the room cool and block out light from street lamps and switch off all lights in the room (even the tiny charging light on an electric toothbrush).
- Studies show that your sleep cycle is set days before so for the best sleep keep each day's routine the same both for you and your baby, including at weekends, as much as possible. Sleep is biologically determined by light levels, hormone cycles, tiredness and so on, so go with both you and your baby's biologically determined sleep patterns, e.g. going to bed perhaps much earlier than you are used to and getting up earlier. This might mean leaving 'jobs' unfinished from the night before, and instead completing them in the morning when you are more refreshed. Going outside with your baby and walking in the morning is really important in setting melatonin levels to help you both sleep that night. Make sure you are not hungry. Keep light levels low with no screens during nighttime as these put the brain on alert. Keep your mobile phone out of your bedroom even if it is switched off as this puts your brain into an alert 'social' state rather than the one required for sleep.
- We need to feel psychologically and physically safe to sleep, both as a baby and as a parent. When we have a baby, this will extend to feeling sure the baby is safe too. Notice if you feel any unease, or are on any alert, e.g. about yourself, your partner, or whoever is sharing a room with you or your baby. See if you can work out what would settle this unease. Use your compassionate mind to help with this.
- Notice if there is anything else that might be creating worry, e.g. not quite trusting that the last one to bed remembered to lock the doors. See what could help to settle any such worries. Use your compassionate mind to help notice and to problem-solve.
- Uncertainty, not just threat, is linked to a lack of safeness, so notice whether there is anything that you need to create more certainty about, e.g. having clear information about when your partner or other family members will be returning home at night, a clear plan around who is 'on duty' to look after your baby when you go to sleep and that you feel happy about how they will carry out this care. Anything else that may be going around in your mind that can be settled for you? A large trigger for uncertainty is not knowing when your baby will wake in the night, so knowing that for some of each night somebody else will be responding to and feeding your baby can be a powerful way of ensuring good chunks of nourishing sleep.
- Having someone 'on guard' for periods of time at night so you don't have to be: this is thought to be something from our evolutionary heritage, where somebody would be on guard so the rest of the group could sleep.

- Baby looked after elsewhere so brain can go off guard – often parents are still hypervigilant to the possibility their child might wake even whilst they are asleep so no deep sleep can happen unless the baby is cared for by a trusted person elsewhere.
- Our babies have evolved to be close by and to be fed frequently in the early days, so have a set-up where your baby can be responded to quickly and can be reassured by your closeness.
- Associate your bed with sleep rather than being awake. If you are still awake in bed after about twenty minutes then go and sit quietly somewhere else, just doing something relaxing, perhaps some breathing, listening to calming music, or reading an enjoyable book. Only return to bed once you feel sleepy.
- Research has demonstrated three key factors associated with better sleep for mothers and for babies: a calm pre-bedtime routine, a predictable routine and going to bed early.
- Don't try to solve worries in the night. The pre-frontal cortex needed to solve problems isn't so active so we can't problem-solve effectively at night. It can help to write the worry on a pad of paper next to you, so you know you won't forget it. Ask others to help you solve worries with you during the day. Switch systems so that you are in your compassionate mind and out of your threat when you come to problem-solve your worries, as the compassionate mind brings online the part of the brain involved in problem-solving.
- Feed the baby in a place that is set up to be comfortable and pleasant for you. Make sure you can position yourself and your baby comfortably in an optimal position for you to feed and for your baby to be fed. For example, lying slightly back but not flat with baby's tummy to your tummy stimulates many reflexes in the baby which help them to feel safe and better able to breastfeed. Sometimes mothers end up in a more hunched over position as they try to 'do it right' which inadvertently stimulates threat systems rather than safeness systems needed for feeding. Ask for advice from your health visitor or breastfeeding organisations about this. If you are bottle feeding, make sure the whole process from start to finish can be set up so it is as efficient and enjoyable as possible. Set your environment up so you like being there – perhaps having relaxing smells, pictures, textures – anything to help you feel taken care of. Ensure you can feel the right temperature. Have a drink of water nearby. If you have to go into another room, for example to prepare a bottle, see if it is possible to turn it into a pleasant 'nighttime mode', for example with a dim but useable light, a nice smell and sounds that you can just switch on for that moment.
- There is huge variation in the amount a new baby wakes and sleeps; however, research has found that the more we view our baby's waking as 'normal' the better we deal with it, even if they are waking frequently.
- Research is showing that an important trigger for sleep is 'sleep pressure', which is how tired we feel. So just be aware that if you do manage to get to sleep, perhaps while the baby is asleep during the day, then the brain may take longer to allow you to sleep that night. Short naps during the day though are important in terms of mental and physical health and won't affect sleep pressure.

End of practice.

Practice: Compassionate mind for sleep

This is designed to feel like a gentle lullaby so that you could use it yourself, or with your child (when they are old enough) to prepare you both for bed. (Although your baby will enjoy the rhythm and intonation of your voice and feel of your body too even if they can't understand the words.)

- Lie down in your bed with your eyes closed or your gaze resting gently on an object. Bring a warmth, softness and kindness to your face and to your voice. You might welcome yourself here, 'Hello'.
- Imagine you are lying on a cloud. Let your body sink into its softness, letting it hold you and support you.
- Breathe in, and slowly breathe out. In your mind you might say slowly and with warmth, 'I am breathing in; I am breathing out'.
- The cloud lifts up and takes you on a journey. Notice what you can see as you fly snug and warm on your cloud. It takes you to a wonderful place, where you feel totally at ease and free. A place where you can fully breathe out. A place where you can be just as you need to be.
- Notice what you can see in this place. The colours, the light, what is here in this place?
- 'What can I see? What can I see?'
- Tune in to what you can hear. Closer sounds, more distinctive sounds. Then behind those you might tune in to quieter sounds, farther away sounds.
- 'What can I hear? What can I hear?'
- Tune in to what you can touch, and the feel of the air on your skin. It all feels just right.
- 'What can I touch? What can I touch?'
- Notice the smells in this place. Then behind those, you might notice more delicate smells.
- 'What can I smell? What can I smell?'

- Feel the rhythm of your breathing as you settle in to this place.
- 'I am breathing in. I am breathing out'.
- This place is your place. It is here just for you. It is glad that you are here.
- 'Hello place. Hello place.'
- Notice how you are in this place. What do you do? You are free to do whatever you wish.
- You may decide to rest in this place or to return home on your cloud.
- Enjoy the feeling of resting, of settling, of feeling held, supported.
- 'I am settling down. I am settling down.'
- Allow your breath to slow.
- Saying more slowly and with warmth and gentleness 'I am b r e a t h i n g in . . . I am b r e a t h i n g out . . .'
- Just allow yourself to be.

End of practice.

Practice: Compassionate mind for you as you prepare your baby for sleep

- Settle comfortably near to where your baby will be placed to sleep. You may wish to stand so you can walk and move with your baby or settle into where you feed your baby at night.
- Make sure you are warm and comfortable.
- Settle into your sense of steadiness and calm.
- Bring your warm, kind face and your warm, kind voice to this practice.

- You may wish to say in your mind, or out loud with warmth; 'Hello baby, hello baby.'
- 'Here we are. Here we are.'
- Feel the warmth and weight of your baby in your arms.
- Imagine a warm, soft light or colour, perhaps of joy and love or calm, or a whisper, or wish of joy and love or calm, or kindness, or whatever you wish to send to your baby, flowing out of your body and into your baby.
- Allow your breath to slow down – 'We are breathing in. We are breathing out.'
- You might make the sound of the sea as you breathe out ('ocean breathing'), as if you are fogging your glasses or a mirror to clean them but with your mouth more closed. Making the sound long and slow. Breathing in, then ocean breathing out again. Enjoying the long, slow rhythm. Enjoy sharing the rhythm with your baby. Perhaps swaying gently with the rhythm.
- You might hum to your baby, long, slow and deep. Notice the feel of the hum in your chest.
- Notice the feel of the hum passing into your baby.
- Breathe in, then slowly and deeply hum once again.
- You might move or sway with your baby as you hum.
- Feel your steadiness, your strength, your ability to bring this willingness to being with your baby, however they are, however you are, for as long as is needed, and for as many times as is needed. Your warm, wise, kind, compassionate mind. Bringing this gift to your baby, of helping them to sleep.
- 'I am here. I am here.'
- Repeat this practice as many times as you need.

End of practice.

Practice: A mini compassionate mind practice for when you hear your baby wake

- 'Body like a mountain' (even if just getting out of bed).
- 'Breath like the wind.'
- 'Mind like the clear blue sky.'
- Warm, kind face, and warm, kind voice (imagine saying 'Hello' with warmth to yourself first and then to your baby).
- Then imagine filling your whole body up with warmth and a compassionate light as you get up and walk to get your baby. Enjoy the feeling of this as you walk and as you move.
- Then imagine the warmth and compassionate light flowing out of your arms and body into your baby.

End of practice.

Write here your plans or notes for what you intend to put in place to help with sleep.

My sleep notes/plan for me:

____

____

____

____

____

____

____

____

e.g.:

- *Go out with baby every day even in rain to get the light levels to help sleep at night.*
- *Talk to partner about the things that go round in my head at night that stop me sleeping, even the 'silly' things.*
- *Get a warm dressing gown for when I get up to the baby.*
- *What else do I need to feel settled and comfortable at night when I am feeding my baby?*

My sleep notes/plan for my baby:

____

____

____

____

____

____

____

____

e.g.

- *Go out for walk every day to help melatonin levels and set sense of day and night for them.*
- *Create more calm in the evenings by:*

  ____

  ____

  ____

  ____

- *Create a predictable routine that is specific to night-time sleeping, e.g. bath, dress in specific night-time sleep clothes, read them a book, give them milk. All in a place where they will sleep for the night:*

  ____

  ____

  ____

  ____

- *Take up Mum on offer for baby to sleep at hers for one night a week – work out plan for this.*

Our family sleep notes/plan:

____

____

____

____

____

____

____

e.g.:

- *For these early weeks after having baby (won't be for long in scheme of things), me to go to bed with baby.*
- *Loose plan: dinner together as family.*
- *Write notes to share with each other on 'family pad' so can jot them down when we're apart and not forget them.*
- *Have bath with baby straight after dinner.*

- *Partner to dry baby off and get them ready for bed while I finish bath and get ready for bed.*
- *Me feed baby and read them book.*
- *Partner clears up kitchen.*
- *Make commitment with partner to meet together for breakfast in morning even if only ten minutes.*
- *Make notes on 'family pad' if not had time to discuss all wanted to.*

Reflections and notes: What would you like to take hold of and remember from this section about sleep? What would you like to take forward and try? What might be your next steps?

____

____

____

____

____

Section 5:

Creating a secure attachment for our baby (and for ourselves)

Module 26: Secure base and safe haven

Secure base

As we develop our compassionate mind, we are creating a brain and body pattern that is helpful to us in particular and powerful ways. These include creating a feeling of safeness within us, and a sense of strength, confidence and encouragement. It enables us to become more creative in our thinking and problem-solving, and switches on the part of the brain that is involved in learning and integrating new information. And because we are so strongly wired to be social, and to have an imagination, we develop a relationship with our own compassionate mind just as we would with a real person. This of course is the same for our inner self-critic.

Our compassionate mind acts as our own internal attachment figure. In many ways it is like having our own ideal parent, partner, champion or coach inside of us. To be an inner figure that can support us, encourage us and settle us when we feel overwhelmed is quite a skill. In fact, it requires a whole raft of skills. These are the same skills that we need as parents. So, as we learn to develop our compassionate mind, we are learning how to become skilful parents, and vice versa.

This section is all about the micro skills that we need as parents that help form the bedrock of our children's minds and mental and physical health. It prepares them for life and the social world. It also helps them to develop their own compassionate mind that they can then use to help themselves and others. These are also the micro skills that we need to develop and use our compassionate mind in relation to ourselves and others.

Two key aspects we develop in relation to our baby (and also in relation to ourselves and others) is becoming their secure base and their safe haven. The secure base is the sense of a steady presence that they can trust in and rely on. It is a predictable safe presence, who guides, scaffolds new learning so that it is challenging but not too hard, but who also brings a joy, delight and playfulness to this exploration and discovery. Having us as their secure presence means that they are able to move out into the world, play, explore, learn and engage with it when we are with them. In three circles terms, we would be in our drive (blue) and soothing (green) system with perhaps a little bit of threat (red) if we are being encouraged to face something that is a little bit challenging for us. It means that, over time with a secure base, we can develop the skills of wisdom, courage and commitment. All key for living well and the development of the compassionate mind.

A secure base gives us courage and confidence. Imagine you are going somewhere new, and you feel a bit anxious about it. Perhaps you are going to the parent and baby group for the first time. You get a text from your partner or a good friend who just says 'Good luck. Hope you get on well.' Just knowing you are held in mind by somebody can help you, can give you enough confidence to go in, even though it is still scary. It can be much harder to do it alone.

When you get in to the parent and toddler group, your baby might sit on your lap and just take it all in.

If you were to suddenly put them on the floor at this point, what might happen?

____

____

____

They might get distressed and want to be picked up again then sit much closer to you. Your presence then settles them, and they might begin to look around again. They might then want to get down or to explore something with you. Knowing you are a kind, understanding, predictable, steady presence will give them confidence over time. They also see your delight when they are able to master something difficult, so this conditions positive feelings about exploration, learning and dealing with challenges.

We might worry that our baby will become 'clingy' or dependent upon us unless we push them to do things without us. In fact, the opposite is true; the more secure they feel with us, the more independent and confident they will eventually become.

They might need some encouragement occasionally whilst being supported and 'scaffolded' by us.

When have you noticed yourself using your secure base over the last week or so?

Who are the people that act as your secure base at the moment? (There may be one person, or different people according to what you are trying to do.)

How did you use them? Did you see them, phone them, imagine their voice, bring up a memory of them?

Have you noticed yourself being your own secure base? How did you do this? (You might become aware of words of encouragement that you give yourself, or when you broke something down into steps in your mind to make it easier for yourself – 'scaffolding' – for example.)

How does your baby use their secure base? (e.g. They might pull somebody's hand to get them to pick up a toy for them, or look around at the world while in your arms, or reach out to someone from the arms of their secure base person, or point at objects for you to name.)

____

____

____

Safe haven

When we go out into the world, things may go wrong. We might get scared or upset or hurt. Then we need to return to the person who is our secure base, but this time we need them to do something quite different. Rather than teaching us, encouraging us, playing with us, or making us a bit excited about what we might learn, do and find, they will be a pair of welcoming arms and they will settle and soothe us, and help us to become regulated again. They act as a 'safe haven' like a safe harbour in a storm that we can come back to. Their presence, words, touch, voice, understanding, bring a pattern of safeness to our threat system. This does all sorts of things including releasing hormones, activating our vagus nerve, activating memories and the bodily feelings associated with them; a highly complicated cascade of body and brain activity that forms the soothing/safeness system. We have been wired through millions of years of evolution to have our threat systems settled by social safeness. As our soothing/safeness system gets stimulated we begin to calm back down and will eventually move back into a pattern of soothing and safeness ourselves. This is what we see when our baby becomes scared and turns to the person who is their safe haven. They then calm, and eventually get to a pattern in their body and mind where they can then look out or move back out into the world again.

As we get older we can 'internalise' our secure base and safe haven. This is where we might not necessarily need the physical presence of them, but can use our memory of them to think 'what might . . . say or do now?' We can also be really helped by a phone call or a text. Despite all of this, the fastest regulator is still often the physical presence of the person who is our secure base and safe haven, no matter how old we get. Which is why the loss of somebody even when we are 'grown up' can feel like it has pulled the floor out from under us. No matter how much we know with absolute certainty that they will die, we have still lost our secure base and safe haven.

Who acts as your safe haven at the moment? (There may be different people for different settings.)

How do they help you?

Have you noticed yourself being your own safe haven? What do you do for yourself that helps?

How has your baby used their safe haven over the last few days?

Reflections and notes: What would you like to take hold of and remember from this section about secure base and safe haven? What would you like to take forward and try? What might be your next steps?

____

____

____

____

____

Module 27: A secure attachment

We have seen how the process of pregnancy changes the maternal brain. These changes interact with oxytocin which increases during pregnancy and labour. Together these brain and hormonal changes not only produce maternal caregiving behaviours but help co-ordinate them with the infant's mental and behavioural state in a sensitive, attuned and responsive manner. This then all comes together to help the infant to develop a secure attachment.

A secure attachment is where a person feels settled and reassured in the presence of their attachment figure (often a parent or family member, or other people who regularly care for the baby). Later, teachers, friends and then our partner can become attachment figures. When a person is securely attached, they can trust in and use the presence of that attachment figure to give themselves confidence in doing difficult things. Through experience they develop the memories and the knowledge that this person would be willing to help them, and would be able to settle and soothe them when they feel upset or overwhelmed. In three circles terms, a securely attached child experiences their attachment figure as the 'eyes and ears' looking out for danger for them so that they don't have to, and instead can be in their safeness/soothing system. This means that they are then freed up to be able to play, learn and explore, so developing a flourishing drive system too. But if danger does come, then the child has learned that this person will protect them from the danger, deal with the danger and be able to settle them back down again.

Although the brain changes that occur during and after pregnancy give enormous help in terms of parenting, these skills can also be learned. Mothers who have not experienced the same degree of brain changes, or those who have not given birth, such as adoptive parents, or partners of the person who has given birth, or other people closely involved in the care of the baby, can all become sensitive, attuned, secure attachment figures for the baby.

Even those who have had a difficult start to their relationship with their baby, perhaps through experiencing depression or psychosis, separation from their baby perhaps through serious ill health of themselves and/or the baby, birth trauma, or their own early trauma, can build secure, sensitive attachment relationships. However, these early months and years are so crucial to our baby that it is particularly important that parents receive early treatment for anxiety and depression. This is why so much funding has been going in to developing services to help parents with mental health difficulties. So do seek help as early as possible if you are struggling.

Our partner and other involved people will also be developing their own relationship with our child. These relationships are going to differ; for example, the mother is likely to relate to her baby in a different way to the father. The differences are important in helping our child to develop different areas of their brain, physiology and behaviour. Access to other caregivers apart from the mother therefore is important in 'growing' a versatile, resilient, well-rounded child. They can also provide another source of secure attachment for our child while we are recovering physically and mentally, for example from childbirth or mental illness, or even if we are just busy or tired. As we have seen earlier in the book, humans are set up to have multiple people involved in the care of their baby. Sadly, in many societies, parents often parent with very little other help. What is tragic, is that if we struggle, many of us might believe it is because of a failing on our part as a parent, rather than the fact that bringing up a human baby requires support beyond two parents. The message is therefore to get help and support as early as possible, to not feel like the mother is supposed to be the entirety of a child's world; the 'village' is key for our child's development. Once we have recovered, we can then resume learning these skills more intensively and can come back together and reconnect more fully with our baby, where the relationship with them can catch up.

It is never too late to work on our relationship with our children (or anyone actually, including ourselves).

When our baby is born, we become acutely aware of how totally dependent they are upon us for their survival. Luckily, evolution sets up a whole set of behaviours and motivational systems in both the parent and the baby to help this process. The mother will have already had her maternal care-giving system primed by brain changes and hormones of pregnancy and birth. The baby will also be primed too. We always need to hold in mind that there are many individual differences in this, on both the part of the mother and the baby, and that many changes take place after birth too, in the brains of the baby, mother and any other involved caregivers. Here we are looking at the broad picture of what evolution sets up in the mother and the baby.

These are some of the behaviours we have evolved as humans to use with our baby:

- Wanting to hold and have physical proximity to them.
- Gazing at our baby's face and body.
- Talking in 'motherese' or 'infant directed talk'. (This is where we find ourselves speaking more slowly, in a varied, exaggerated, musical manner, repeating words and phrases. Babies prefer this way of being spoken to and it makes learning easier for them.)
- Expression of positive feelings towards the baby.
- Affectionate touch such as stroking their skin, kissing their head, putting our finger in their hand so they can hold it.
- Breathing in the smell of our baby.
- We also immediately begin responding in a social way – so having 'conversations', which even a very young baby will join in with. As you speak to your newborn you might notice that they move an arm or a leg or move their head in response. Then they pause, waiting for you to talk again, then their body will respond again. (Unlike an adult, the newborn can only engage in this for the briefest of moments before they will need to look away as that is a lot of stimulation for their new brain.)

What from this list have you and others been drawn to do in relation to your baby? (Carry this exercise out from your compassionate mind, particularly if you are feeling tired, overwhelmed or critical of yourself.)

____

____

____

____

____

____

Anything else not on this list?

We also see that our baby is born already primed with a set of behaviours, including:

- Wanting to be physically close to us
- Wanting to feed for nourishment and for comfort
- Wanting to be physically held
- Wanting to be talked to in positive and affectionate tones
- Preferring our voice and smell to a stranger's
- Preferring 'motherese' (infant directed talk)
- Wanting interactions that are sensitive, synchronous (in time with) and attuned (matched with their needs and intentions)

So quite incredibly, both the parent *and* the baby are primed to begin a social relationship with each other as soon as the baby is born (but possibly even whilst the baby is in the womb too).

What from this list do you notice your baby is drawn to? What do they seem to prefer? What seems to settle them?

Anything else not on this list?

Our baby is dependent on physical contact and care-giving behaviours for the maturation of their brain and body systems essential for social interaction. These behaviours have an impact on our baby's brain, hormones, body and behaviour. Our interactions are setting up our baby to develop a secure attachment and be able to skilfully navigate the complex social world of humans. It is thought that our success as humans is due to our sophisticated social brain which enables us to quickly identify and mentally share the emotional states of others. As we interact with our baby, we are laying the foundations for them to be able to successfully manage being part of human life. Such skills will include developing this ability to understand the minds of others, to be able to regulate the emotional states of themselves and others, and to work with others towards a goal.

When we are interacting in this way with our baby, we are laying down in them the hormonal, brain and body signatures of what it is to feel safe. So, right from the time when our baby is in the womb, they are developing a brain and body that form the foundation of their compassionate brain.

Even though our newborn infant will only be interacting with us for a few moments throughout the day, these interactions will be powerful and long lasting in terms of creating lifelong patterns.

We will be looking in more detail at these interactions. The intention is not to place pressure on us to be constantly trying to interact with our baby in perfectly minded, synchronised, sensitive and attuned ways. In fact, studies have shown that we only need to be 'getting it right' or roughly right, for about a third of our interactions. (This doesn't of course mean we can be shouting at our baby or completely ignoring them for two-thirds of the time. It is more about trying to do the best we can all of the time, but it really doesn't need to be perfection.) If we feel under pressure, then we will have moved into the threat pattern of our mind, rather than the soothing/safeness system, and it is the soothing/safeness system that underpins the behaviours that we are talking about. Instead, the intention is to highlight how incredible these tiny interactions are and to become consciously aware of what we are probably doing subconsciously. This then helps us to identify when we have gone off track with our interactions, and to know just what 'getting back on track again' looks like. This section is all about a light touch, a dance, a playfulness, having a go, something that is filled with ease and warmth – so in other words, triggered off, and held, by our compassionate mind.

As we and our baby learn how to relate to each other, the brain waves, hormones, body and behaviour of each become synchronised (attuned to and regulated by one another). By just three months after being born, this parent-infant synchrony can predict the child's cognitive, social and emotional skills across early childhood. What might seem unimportant, or 'just playing', is actually forming a foundation for our child's ability to manage their own emotional and physiological state, and to be able to form relationships with others.

Reflections and notes: What would you like to take hold of and remember from this section about secure attachment? What would you like to take forward and try? What might be your next steps?

____

____

____

____

Module 28: Neurodivergence, temperament and developmental differences with regard to attachment and parenting

We may be an autistic parent, or have an autistic child, or perhaps both. We and/or our baby may have other developmental differences. Perhaps our baby was born prematurely or very poorly and spent time on a neonatal unit. We may have a very different temperament to our baby; perhaps we are very sensitive to noise and stimulation and prefer the quiet company of others, but our baby relishes stimulation and lots of different people.

These differences might mean that how our baby communicates with us or what makes them feel settled and safe is quite different from what we expect or are familiar with. Our baby might also be different from other children that we are used to.

It might make parenting our baby a little trickier, at least initially, but often just means that we might take longer to get to know our baby and therefore need to give ourselves and our baby the extra time that is needed. The importance of trying to understand our baby's mind, doing our best to respond moment to moment to them, and responding with warmth and care, still all apply. It is all about getting to know *our* baby but also working out what helps us to parent at our best too – so we are getting to know ourselves as a parent too. For example, some autistic mothers described how they took a while to feel bonded to their baby because they required the kind of feedback that comes from an older baby in order for the bond to develop. They also developed strategies such as choosing quieter toys to have in their house and leaving more stimulating toys at, say, Grandma's house. They chose social contact carefully and went to activities that both they and their baby enjoyed together. They also set up strategies with regard to sensitivity to smell, such as manageable ways to change nappies that smelled aversive and leaving the feeding of food they struggled with for when their partner could feed it to them.

(There are now a growing number of websites and support groups being set up to help parents such as those who are autistic, have ADHD or highly sensitive personalities, who might find aspects of parenting challenging. They often have some really helpful suggestions.)

As we will see, mind-mindedness, synchrony, maternal bonding, and parent-infant attachment flow from safeness. So, the key for parent and baby is to establish that safeness for them *both*.

What do you struggle with in terms of parenting at the moment that may be to do with your particular brain set-up or personality?

____

____

What helped you before you had a baby?

____

____

____

____

____

____

What might help you with these aspects now?

____

____

____

____

____

____

> *Mind-mindedness, synchrony, maternal bonding, and parent infant attachment all flow from safeness.*
>
> *So, the key for parent and baby is to establish that safeness for them both.*

Reflections and notes: What would you like to take hold of and remember from this section about neurodivergence, temperament and developmental differences? What would you like to take forward and try? What might be your next steps?

Module 29: The different behavioural states of our newborn

Before we look at the micro skills that we use in interactions, it can be helpful to be able to notice the different states that our baby can be in. Our baby will constantly move through these different states (as do we) but will spend different amounts of time in them as they develop. Some babies move more slowly between them, others more quickly. Knowing the different behaviours indicating each state will give us clues as to how to be with our baby in each state and how to pick the optimal states for particular things such as playing with our baby. This also helps us to know when we need to change what we are doing if they are becoming more upset, in order to help them come back to a calm state. In compassionate mind terms we are helping to keep our baby out of threat and instead helping them in moving between the drive and soothing/safeness system according to what our baby is 'telling' us they need or want.

The different behavioural states of our newborn

In newborns, Dr T.B. Brazelton (a paediatrician who worked extensively with newborns) identified six behavioural states:

Deep sleep (State 1): the baby is still and quiet with eyes shut. They may stir but stay asleep. This is where memories are laid down.

Light sleep (State 2): the baby's eyes can be seen 'fluttering' and moving about under the eyelids. Breathing will be quick and shallow. The baby might make all sorts of little noises and facial expressions.

Drowsy (State 3): the baby's eyes may open and close, but they are not focused on anything. Breathing is faster than in deep sleep. There is a lot of movement in arms and legs. They might wake up fully or go back into deep sleep. They are sensitive to stimuli in this state and might be able to be soothed back to sleep or woken up fully.

Quiet alert (State 4): the baby is aware of and engaged with their surroundings but is at ease and in a calm state just taking in information, playing, exploring or interacting socially. They will respond to us, and this is the best state for playing with our baby and for feeding them.

Alert and active (State 5): the baby is on their way to crying. Their movements become jerkier and they may lose focus on the stimuli. They are sensitive to stimuli and there is still a possibility of distracting the baby, changing position or activity and calming them back down again.

Crying (State 6): the baby cries and may move into more distressed crying. They will not be receptive to new information or stimuli and are unlikely to be helped by being distracted. Instead, they need the caregivers to act quickly to resolve the issue and to cuddle and soothe them until they move back into the quiet alert state. The baby may be crying because they are hungry or tired but will need to be settled back down to a quieter state before they can feed or sleep. They may only be receptive to being held and receiving gentle, rhythmic, familiar stimuli such as gentle jigging and patting, and soothing repetitive vocal sounds. This is the state that is most effective at attracting the attention of caregivers.

In compassionate mind terms the quiet alert state is a response to being in the safeness/soothing system. All is well and there is nothing that they need. This is where they might move more into their drive system by indicating an activity, trying an activity that you suggest, or wanting you to follow and respond to where their interest takes them. This is the state in which they can explore and learn. Alert and active (State 5) and crying (State 6) are what we see when they are moving into the threat system.

Which of the above states has your baby been in so far today?

____

____

____

____

____

Which states would you say you have been in so far today? (These are of course not meant to be used for adults, but we can relate to these states too.)

____

____

____

____

____

Reflections and notes: What would you like to take hold of and remember from this section about different behavioural states? What would you like to take forward and try? What might be your next steps?

____

____

____

____

____

Module 30: Mind-mindedness

In order to interact with our baby, we need to be able to tell whether our interactions are helping them or upsetting them. This may sound obvious, but often our baby gives out only smalls signals as to how they are feeling. If we are too eager or too in threat ourselves then we can miss or misinterpret these signals. We need to set out with the intention of trying to learn what our baby is telling us. This will get easier over time as our baby develops and we learn more about them. This intention of getting to know our baby's mind is called 'mind-mindedness'.

Mind-mindedness is our ability to treat our children as individuals with their own mind as separate from our own, with their own thoughts and feelings. It involves paying attention to what our baby might be thinking or feeling and then responding appropriately. For example, for a baby that is reaching for a teddy, we might say 'Oh you like teddy don't you? You'd like to hold teddy?' and then pass teddy to the baby. Misinterpreting this as the baby wanting to be picked up or saying, 'Looks like it's time for a sleep' for example, would not be mind-mindedness as this is not what is indicated by the baby's behaviour. We may of course get this wrong, but we would then respond to our baby's indication that we had got it wrong. So, if we picked them up thinking they wanted sleep and they are still reaching for the teddy we might correct ourselves and say, 'Oh, you wanted the teddy. I thought you wanted a sleep. Ah, here's teddy.' This is the basis of sensitive and attuned interactions, the 'dance' we have with our baby. It forms the bedrock of many other significant aspects for our baby including the notion that they are being carefully and positively held in mind by us, that they are regarded as important and worthy of care and attention, and that they have their own control and agency in the world. This is how secure attachment develops. It also underpins being able to regulate their own emotions later in life and their ability to understand the minds of others.

Here is another example: we might be playing a game with our baby and then they begin to get upset. Carrying on playing the game to its end because it is our favourite game would not be mind-minded because we are holding ourselves in mind rather than our baby. We might say, 'Oh was that a bit too much? You've had enough of that one then,' then pick them up to soothe them.

Mind-mindedness is therefore not just about noticing our baby's mental state but also making appropriate responses. So, it is the relationship and the interaction, the to and the fro, like a conversation that also involves our bodies.

In fact, more recent research has shown that we demonstrate mind-mindedness not just by the comments we make but how our body responds. For example, if we need to move our baby who is happily playing on their play mat, from one place to another because we are taking them with us into another room, we might approach our baby slowly rather than suddenly, putting our hands out to demonstrate our intention, indicating with our face and our words that we are intending to pick them up, then picking them up gently. We would do this because we understand our baby's mind: that they might experience shock if we were to suddenly bend down and pick them up. This is called parental embodied mentalisation (PEM).

Again, it is our responsivity to the baby's responses that is key, but with PEM we are revealing our understanding of our baby's mind through how we adjust our movement in relation to our baby's non-verbal or verbal signals. For example, if we suddenly brought a toy in fast in front of our baby, and this made the baby pull their body back and put their arms up to block this, how might we respond to this? If we noticed this and then moved the toy back further, bringing it towards them more slowly, all the way paying attention to what their body and voice might be telling us, then this is embodied mentalisation.

Understanding our own baby takes time. When our baby is newborn, we are getting to know them, and they are getting to know us. Research has shown that the cries of young babies do not give information about what they need; they do not have a 'signature' cry for say wanting food, which is different to their cry for wanting company. Instead, it seems that they are crying to signal an undifferentiated feeling of distress. This research showed that parents were making a best guess as to the reason for the cry based on information such as time since the last feed or nappy change. So, we don't need to feel bad that we don't know exactly what they are wanting when our baby cries. What is different is the cry of different babies which changes over age so that we can distinguish our baby's cries from those of another baby. In evolutionary terms this suggests that the aim of a young infant's cry is to alert their own parent as fast as possible to their need for them. The cry stimulates in the parent a need to come fast and to pick the baby up and try to resolve the issue.

In summary, mind-mindedness is about doing our best to connect with our baby and to learn about their specific mind and how to respond accordingly. It is also about being able to notice when we have got it wrong, then repairing that 'rupture' to then connect again. In compassionate mind terms, we are learning what is 'helpful and not harmful' when we are interacting with our baby.

List some examples of mind-mindedness with your baby that you've done recently either verbally or with your body. (Remember to switch into your compassionate mind first to help you notice these):

____

____

____

____

____

____

List some examples of mind-mindedness that you noticed your partner doing recently:

____

____

____

____

____

____

Noticing this helps us to become consciously aware of something that is very skilful but which we may never have noticed that we do. In terms of compassionate attention (see this section later in the book) it is also important to deliberately focus our attention on what is going well and to lay these down as memories and brain changes. We can then draw on these to balance out the times when our threat mind will get hold of us (as it will do), leaving us feeling we are only getting parenting wrong.

When do you find it easier to be mind-minded with your baby?

____

____

____

____

____

____

What makes it harder to be mind-minded with your baby?

____

____

____

____

____

____

You might notice that it is much easier to pay attention to the mind of your baby when you are feeling more settled, rested, fed. In other words when you feel in your safeness/soothing system. You are more likely to find it harder when you are tired, worried, busy, frustrated, hungry, in a rush, in other words, in your threat system. Our ability to be mind-minded is not something that we are necessarily good or bad at (although like any skill we can work to improve it), it is just very sensitive to how under threat or settled and safe we feel (again like most other skills).

This means that we can become better at being mind-minded with our baby by using our compassionate mind training. Of course it is hard to remember to practise, and hard to find the time to practise, particularly when we may even start our day by being woken by our baby. But the implications for ourselves and our baby are far too great for us to discard this.

Instead, we can bring our compassionate mind to the issue of how to practise, to help us come up with solutions, commit to it because it is important to us, and to help ourselves rather than criticise ourselves when we don't do what we had hoped.

Practice: To help with mind-mindedness with your baby

- Shift your posture so that even if you are holding your baby, you feel steady, stable, grounded, feet hip width apart and steady, back upright, shoulders back and down ('dignified' posture, 'body like a mountain').
- Allow your face to soften and loosen and bring a warm, kind smile and voice to yourself and your baby ('Hello [your name]!, Hello [baby's name]!').
- Allow your breathing to become slower. Slowing the in breath, bringing it deep into the base of your lungs, feeling the pause, then really slowing the out breath. You might notice your body becoming steadier as your breathing begins to move into its own soothing rhythm.
- Like a mountain in the midst of the forever changing weather surrounding it, notice your feeling of steadiness, no matter what is happening with your baby.
- Feel yourself stepping into a part of you that has committed to showing up fully for your baby in this moment. You intention is just to be here with your baby, bringing your warm, wise, kind, compassionate mind to them and their mind for these next moments, doing the best you can, working these interactions out together, the two of you.
- Bring a manner of playfulness, curiosity, interest, light and ease. You are here to discover a little more about their mind in this moment, like looking in more detail at a picture or a flower or animal with the intention of just enjoying the discovery and the experience.
- Breathing in. Breathing out, keeping your face, your jaw, your tongue loose and relaxed.
- Notice when an interaction goes wrong with as much interest and warmth and intention to learn as when it goes right.
- Bring to mind a sense of holding both you and your baby with warm understanding, with wisdom, strength and compassion, with a lightness of touch, gently, taking your time.

- Carry on for as long as you wish.
- When you finish this practice see if you can keep the intention of moving into the next few moments in this manner as best you can.

End of practice.

Try doing this practice before or during your interactions with your baby. Compare it to when you haven't done the practice. What do you notice?

____

____

____

____

____

____

Imagine your compassionate other or self was spending time with you, perhaps imagining that they have turned up when you were struggling recently.

- Tune in to how they pay attention to your mind.
- How do they give you the sense that they understand you deeply?
- How do they let you know that they care about you and are committed to helping you?
- What is it that they do or say that enables you to feel safe and confident in their presence?

It might be what they say, or perhaps how they move and interact with you.

____

____

____

____

____

____

For example:

- It might be that they comment on how you seem to be feeling or that they understand why you are feeling this way because they have spent time getting to know your mind; 'You are looking very stressed and anxious about this. I am wondering if this is because you so want to get this right?'
- They may demonstrate their understanding that you don't like close contact by sitting at the distance from you that feels just right for you.
- They may speak in a voice tone that feels safe and comfortable for you.
- If they get things wrong, they notice by paying attention to your reaction, and then trying to repair this as best they can.

Reflections and notes: What would you like to take hold of and remember from this section about mind-mindedness? What would you like to take forward and try? What might be your next steps?

____

____

____

____

____

Module 31: Synchrony

As we use our mind-mindedness skills to enable us to work out as best we can what our baby may be wanting in this moment, we then find that we start to tune into our baby and move in a kind of 'dance' with them. This attuned interaction is called 'synchrony'.

Synchrony occurs during warm, attuned, face-to-face interactions between the parent and the baby, where the parent co-ordinates the rhythm of their interactions with those of their baby. It can be seen in the repetitive, rhythmic games such as 'peek-a-boo' or the 'serve and return' of 'conversations'. It has been found that even newborn babies follow the same rules and rhythms of typical conversations. The baby can be seen to be using their body and vocalisations to 'talk' to the parent (the baby 'serves' an initiative, like serving a ball in tennis). The parent 'receives' the initiative, carefully listening, then responds back ('returns' the initiative, like returning a ball). The baby can be seen to pause their body and vocalisations as they 'receive' the return, listen and then wait for their turn, before replying with vocalisations and/or movement. In synchronous behaviour, both the parent and the baby are experiencing shared, positive feelings such as warmth, pleasure, joy and delight. There is a feeling of ease and flow.

As you interact with your baby, bring your compassionate mind to notice with warmth and interest those brief moments of 'conversation' between you and your baby. How does your baby start off a 'conversation' with you? (It might be a look, a sound, a body movement.)

____

____

____

____

____

Over the last day or so, what are some of their 'serves' (where they initiate a conversation with a sound or body movement) and 'returns' (where they respond to you)?

How do you show your baby that you have 'received' their initiative? How do they know that you got it?

How does your baby show you that they have received your 'return'? How do you know that they got it?

Although it may look on the outside that it is just the behaviour that appears co-ordinated, in fact heart rhythms, oxytocin responses and brain waves become co-ordinated too. These brief but intense social moments have an 'imprinting' effect on the baby's brain, creating the building blocks for stress management and for creating affiliative connections with others throughout life.

Synchrony also provides the foundation for an ability to regulate one's own emotions, and to be able to empathise with and understand the minds of others. And the more we can regulate ourselves and understand the minds of others, the more we can synchronise, and so on.

This synchrony between ourselves and our baby builds over time as we and our baby get to know each other. The 'signature' of this synchrony will differ between each pair or 'dyad', for example between mother and baby, father and baby, grandad and baby, but for each specific person it will become predictable and familiar to our baby. This predictability is part of the foundation of the secure base, where a baby (or adult) feels so safe and regulated by our presence that they can move out from us little by little, explore, play, have courage and try difficult things. They can swap between these different 'signatures' according to their needs, for example seeking out more calming, soothing interactions with mum or more energetic and play-directed interactions with dad. These synchrony 'signatures' between two individuals or 'dyads' become richer and more complex over time, from infancy to adolescence and into adulthood, but still maintain that familiarity and predictability.

But it is not just across the lifespan of one relationship, for example between a mother and her child , that we see this ability to synchronise with another. The synchrony 'signatures' developed in infancy ripple out across all relationships, to friends, romantic relationships, people we work with, and even to strangers in distress or those that we need to collaborate with.

Like the other micro skills that we are talking about in this section, synchrony is much harder when we are exhausted, worried and experiencing mental illness such as postnatal depression. Depression in particular affects the reward pathways (part of the drive system) which are important in experiencing our baby as rewarding, and in being able to engage in synchronous and attuned behaviour. So, it is not our fault if we find ourselves struggling with feeling attuned to our baby on top of having depression, as depression impacts the very systems that make parenting easier for us. This is why we emphasise throughout this book how important early treatment, support and other caregivers are in the perinatal period.

But even with postnatal depression, parents are able to offer their baby sensitive and warm interactions, and often go to great lengths to ensure this. Important new interventions currently being researched by Professor Ruth Feldman and her team, which focused on teaching synchronous behaviours in mothers experiencing depression, are revealing promising early results in improving both synchrony between the parent and infant whilst also alleviating the postnatal depression, even though postnatal depression was not the target.

What does synchrony look like?

- The parent's attention is focused on what the infant is trying to look at.
- Face-to-face attention on the baby as they try to communicate.
- The baby's communication is acknowledged.
- Parent's vocalisations are in 'motherese' vocalisations.
- Affectionate touching of the baby whilst paying close attention to how this is being received – whether to carry on, stop, or change it.
- Expression of positive feelings by the parent.
- Care is safe and calm – the parent is experienced as the external regulator.
- The presence of the parent would be experienced as supportive.
- Interactions are relaxed and not tense; both bodies are at ease.
- Moment by moment flexible adaptations by the parent to changing states in the baby.
- Parent helping the baby to build and maintain positive arousal – may be joy, excitement, interest, curiosity, concentration.
- Parent can flexibly shift across and adapt to baby's changing states.
- There is a smooth, rhythmic quality to the interactions.
- There is 'give and take', 'serve and return' between the parent and baby.

The mother provides a safe, calm and supportive presence, acting as an external regulator for the baby. She also responds to the child's communications and adapts with flexibility across states. She is aiming to settle threat states and promote and maintain positive states. So, she is both steady and flexible. In compassionate mind terms, she is regulating the threat system and returning the infant to drive and soothing/safeness states as appropriate (for example, playing 'peek a boo', or singing with the baby, or showing the baby a new toy stimulating joy and excitement, but then settling the baby if the baby becomes over-aroused). This provides an experience of safeness which is doing many things including building the baby's brain, endocrine system, memories of safeness, and positive beliefs about themselves and others. In time, these experiences will enable the child to begin to regulate their own emotions and possess their own ability to be both steady and flexible as they navigate their social world.

This combination of steadiness and flexibility that we see in the parent-baby interactions is also what we are cultivating as we build our compassionate mind. This is why there is a deliberate focus on creating, from the bottom up (literally from our feet first), a body that is both steady and flexible, in order to create a mind which is both steady and flexible.

We create a posture that is grounded, stable and strong, but also flexes and moves to adapt to whatever life throws at us; just like a mighty oak that also moves in the wind, or a tall building built in an earthquake or tornado zone that has deep foundations but also sways slightly with tremors and high winds.

Practice: Weathering the storm

- Sit back in your chair, with your feet flat on the ground hip width apart.
- Feel the ground underneath your feet.
- Sit upright 'like a mountain' or mighty oak tree with your dignified posture. Bring your shoulders up to your ears then drop them down and back, feeling the space in your chest.
- Close your eyes or allow your gaze to rest lightly on an object.
- Bring your warm, kind face and your warm, kind voice tone to your breath. Perhaps greeting it as if you are really pleased to have come across it – 'Hello breath!'.
- Allow your in breath to slow down, bringing it deep into the base of your lungs, notice the pause, and then allow your out breath to become really slow, gentle and smooth. Perhaps use your 'ocean breathing' where you make the sound of the sea by breathing out through your mouth with your throat constricted. You are aiming for a sound you'd make if you were trying to 'fog' a mirror or pair of glasses for cleaning. This slows down and extends the out breath even more.

- Imagine sitting at the foot of a hill or a mountain with an oak tree nearby. You are sitting as steady as them.
- Notice the sun warming your skin, a breeze moving your hair. You feel steady and settled.
- Now imagine the rain beginning to fall on you. You sit steady as the mountain and oak tree in the rain, breathing smoothly and slowly. You notice any discomfort with calmness and understanding.
- The winds then come, blowing your hair and your clothes. You sit steady as the mountain and oak tree in the wind, noticing from your place of steadiness and understanding, the feel of the wind, and any experiences and thoughts running through you.
- You might feel yourself rock with the strongest gusts of wind; you move with the wind, then bring yourself back to your steady, stable centre. Just observing any thoughts or experiences that arise from this place of steadiness, calm and understanding.
- The sky clears and the sun comes out again. You feel the warm sun drying you and warming you once again. You sit steady, calm and centred.
    - ◊ You might imagine bringing this steadiness; both steady but also flexible and adaptable, to the different 'weather' that your baby feels, and creates in you throughout the day – responsive, calm, steady.
- When you are ready, bring your mind back to the sounds in your room. Bring your attention to the feel of your feet on the floor, perhaps moving your feet. Feel your hands in your lap; perhaps moving them. Feel the chair supporting you. When you are ready, gently open your eyes. As you move into the next part of your day, keep this steadiness and flexibility with you as best you can.

End of practice.

Reflections: What was this practice like for you?

What would you like to remember and take forward from this practice?

Ways of practicing synchrony with your baby

- Deliberately focusing on what connects you to your baby (e.g. both like same music, both not so 'huggy' but like hand massages, both like looking up at leaves in the trees, both been through the birth together, etc.)
- Mirroring baby (e.g. copying what they are doing or saying)
- Dancing together
- Singing together
- Co-creating a painting or picture (e.g. with finger paint – when they make a mark, you add to that mark and so on)
- Co-creating music (e.g. when they bang with a spoon, you bang with your spoon. Then bring in different 'instruments' for you both to use together)
- Singing the same song repeatedly so both learn the next bit and can interact together
- Playing the same game repeatedly

- Establishing joint and predictable beginnings and ends to things (e.g. to start and finish of baby massage, baby yoga, changing nappy, bedtime routine, breast/bottle feeding, etc.)
- Clapping together
- Laughing together
- Being 'silly' with your baby (e.g. copying them playing, laying on the floor looking up at what they see, crawling around the house with them, pulling silly faces with them, singing silly made-up songs to them, splashing in puddles with them, running out in the rain with them, hiding in their camp with them, bringing them under a duvet 'camp' made by your body, making messy paintings with them, glitter and glue, colouring in together)
- Making dough or food together
- Blowing bubbles with baby – later teaching them how to blow bubbles
- Playing in sand tray together
- Using water, bubbles, shaving foam, rice, little toys to co-create scenarios or games with each other
- Clean 'messy' play together (e.g. Ziplock plastic bag with bits of coloured paper, paint or glitter in water so you can 'smoosh' it together. Thick paint on paper covered in clingfilm so can move it about together)
- Using dried rice or oat flakes to pour and stir together using different bowls, jugs and spoons

In the research studies where mothers with postnatal depression were taught how to increase their synchrony with their baby, this was done by videoing their interactions and showing them back the moments of synchrony. This helped the mothers to become consciously aware of what synchronous behaviour looks like, meaning they did even more of it. As mentioned above, incredibly this intervention lifted the mothers out of postnatal depression even though this wasn't the focus.

It seems that there was something about this process, perhaps the positive feedback loop for both mother and infant, which alleviated the depression. Or perhaps it was the mothers seeing what to do and discovering that they already had the skills without having realised it. This is very different to a depressed mind, which will 'video' and replay only the moments that went badly – because this is what a threat mind does. But it shows that even when we are depressed, we can move into a different pattern in our mind and body.

This book of course doesn't come with video feedback, but we can teach ourselves, and others, this process of imagining being the camera that takes these video clips through a compassionate lens. The following exercises help us to practise shifting our attention to these moments of synchrony.

- Settle in to your compassionate self or imagine your compassionate other is here with you.
- You are aware of this kind, warm, strong, wise, caring part of you or them, here to help you with this.
- They are here to notice with their warm, curious, helpful mind, the times when you synchronise your body and mind with your baby.
- There is nothing that you need to do but carry on normally with your baby. They will do all the work quietly in the background, unobtrusively capturing those synchronous moments, which you probably won't believe are happening at all, until they sit down with you and share them with you.
- (You can actually ask somebody you trust, such as your partner, friend or family member, to do this in reality. Videoing, although scary, is the most powerful way of doing this. If not, they could take photos on their phone, or just note down moments.)

What clips of synchrony will your compassionate self or compassionate other show you from the last few hours or day or so? (Remember that your threat mind will tell that there won't be any moments, or that people will see just how rubbish a mother you really are. It is therefore important that the threat mind is just nodded at, just briefly acknowledging its presence, then you turn back to your compassionate mind to do this for you. You might need to do this a few times. This is normal.)

____

The aim of this is to see what you are actually doing already, and to make it easier to do even more of it. Then, as you go forwards, you can actively notice when these moments are happening and take them in. This will be changing your brain as well as your baby's. Hopefully, it will be building your positive mental state too.

Parents are likely to have different synchrony patterns or signatures to each other. For example, research has shown that mothers' synchronous behaviour is often more care-focused, more focused on each other, more low and medium arousal building, moves more gently to positive affect, with more face-to-face interactions and affectionate touch. Whereas fathers' patterns of synchrony were, on the whole, more focused on exploration, play, with sudden peaks of positive affect, more focused on the environment, and with more stimulatory contact.

Settle into your compassionate mind and observe those moments of synchrony between your partner and your baby. You might want to actually video these or take photos of these moments, or note them down, then share them with your partner.

What examples did you find over a day or so?

____

____

____

____

____

In what way were their patterns of synchrony similar or different to yours?

____

____

____

____

____

What was it like for you as you took note of them? Did this change over the course of the time you spent consciously noticing? If so, in what way?

____

____

____

____

____

What was it like to share these video clips, photos, notes with your partner?

____

____

____

____

____

There is evidence that not only do we and our baby, and our partner and our baby, begin to synchronise our behaviour and mind over time, but we synchronise with each other as parents too.

- As ever, the threat mind will pick out all the difficult moments between ourselves and our partner, particularly in this intense time of learning, exhaustion and juggling that comes with new parenthood.
- Just note any presence of our threat mind or critic. Maybe give it a nod in acknowledgment, then shift your attention to moving into your compassionate mind.
- ('Body like a mountain, breath like the wind, mind like the sky', warm, kind face and voice, intention to being helpful as best you can, using the wisdom and strength acquired over your whole lifetime).

- Now make an intention or set regular reminders to record moments of synchrony between you and your partner, moments when you feel connected and seem to be working together, interacting smoothly, noticing and sharing each other's minds and emotions, and experiencing feelings of joy and ease in those moments.

Note here what you saw in that period of noticing synchrony between the two of you:

What was that experience like, of noticing synchrony between you?

What was that experience like when you shared what you noticed with your partner?

Reflections and notes: What would you like to take hold of and remember from this section about synchrony? What would you like to take forward and try? What might be your next steps?

____

____

____

____

Module 32: How to prime mind-mindedness and synchrony

1) Physical proximity and touch

As already mentioned, these skills of synchrony and mind-mindedness can be affected by all sorts of things that are not our fault, such as threat, postnatal depression, exhaustion, trauma and so on. We can sometimes get into a negative cycle with our baby, for example where we become reluctant to do the physical care or comfort of our baby because we seem to be getting it wrong or feel unconfident, and we leave this more and more to our partner or mother. Unfortunately, this has biological as well as psychological feedback loops for both us and our baby, where the oxytocin stimulated by physical closeness and touch begins to drop away for both and instead gets associated with the other person that is doing the close care instead. Oxytocin is a key regulator of our maternal behaviour, our brain and our ability to understand our baby's mind (mind-mindedness) and synchronise with our baby. It also helps us and our baby to feel calmer and more settled.

So even though our instinct might be to let others care for our baby, in fact we need to increase physical proximity and touch with our baby in order to stimulate oxytocin, which will then make the other interactions and maternal care easier.

When physical proximity and touch feel hard

Being in physical contact with another person is one of our earliest experiences. We will have very strong body memories of physical contact and touch from a young age. These body memories are carried with us and can be triggered off when we are in similar circumstances of touch and physical closeness. If physical touch and closeness bring up memories of safeness, warmth, feeling snug, feeling settled and calm, of pleasure, then we are likely to seek out physical contact and to want to offer it to others. But what if it wasn't pleasant, or if it was absent? How might we feel in our body when we are in experiences of physical touch and closeness again? We may also have had later experiences of discomfort or harm from touch or closeness. If touch and closeness were registered in our body and mind as harmful, unpleasant or alien then we are likely to develop conscious or unconscious ways of making sure we don't get harmed again. These are called safety strategies, and we will be looking at them in more detail in the section on formulation.

Examples of our safety strategies might be 'keep people at a distance', 'appear scary so people don't come close', 'become overweight so people are less likely to want a physical relationship with me', 'use drugs, medication or alcohol in circumstances where I'm likely to be touched so I can't feel it so much'.

When we become pregnant, give birth and have our baby, suddenly we cannot avoid physical touch and closeness. Even strangers might come and touch our pregnant belly. How do we manage all of this?

We may have had experiences where we felt we were 'bad' or 'harmful' in some way. Again, these can arise from early experiences, for example where we were shamed or given the impression that our behaviour or emotions were harmful to our parents or siblings. (We will look at this in more detail later in the book.) We may develop safety strategies where we keep people at a distance or avoid physical closeness with people we care about because of an (often unconscious) fear that we might harm them. Now we have a baby who is precious to us, and we may be terrified at some level that somehow our 'badness' will harm them, or that if they get close to us, they will somehow suddenly become aware of our 'badness'. So, we keep them physically at a distance to protect them from ourselves.

We can also feel disgusted by physical contact, perhaps through early experiences, or we can feel overwhelmed and overstimulated by physical contact because of our neurobiological set-up or early experiences. Physical examinations, birth, breastfeeding, bathing and holding our baby can feel physically aversive, so we might, perhaps even without realising it, allow others to do more and more of the physical care of our baby.

These experiences are so painful and so sad. They may take us by surprise when we have a baby, especially if we have unconsciously protected ourselves for years by avoiding physical closeness. The more we become consciously aware of our struggles and can see these as our safety strategies designed to keep us safe following experiences or brain/body set-ups that we never chose and are not our fault, then the more we can find ways through with our baby. Both they, and we, are wired to be settled and soothed by physical proximity and touch, so it will be an important ingredient to bring into their life and ours. It is certainly worth the work. But this kind of work is, of course, scary, unpleasant and difficult. It therefore requires our compassionate mind (with its wisdom, warmth, understanding, non-judgement, strength, courage and wish to help us) to be with us as we try as best we can to address this.

Before moving on, spend a moment doing a compassionate self, compassionate other/image or compassionate place practice. Then read on but keep your compassionate mind with you. You might just read with a lightness of touch, letting it wash over you, but allow it to be there even in the background rather than skip it. Allow it to take a place in the life of you and your baby with a commitment to keep revisiting it, particularly as you build your compassionate mind. It may be that you might want to seek help around this (there are now parent-infant services that are particularly helpful) or talk it over with your partner or health visitor.

Reflection: What would you like to take hold of and remember from this? How might you want to take this forward? What might you find helpful?

Ways of increasing physical proximity and touch

- Compassionate systematic desensitisation to closeness, i.e. working up from closeness that is easier to closeness that is harder
- Asking others to do care for your baby that requires touching their skin (but working towards this yourself) whilst finding ways of still holding them, e.g. when they are in their sleepsuit, wrapped in a towel after bathtime, when in outdoor clothing, e.g. their snowsuit or coat
- Holding baby when asleep
- Smelling baby
- Stroking baby's hair
- Putting baby cream on baby's hand
- Putting hand on baby when baby is asleep
- Reading to baby
- Singing to baby

- Dancing gently with baby
- Activities where you are in physical proximity but not so focused on this, e.g. reading to baby with baby next to you rather than on you, watching a programme together, doing messy play next to each other
- Having baby in sling
- Having baby in a baby back carrier
- Baby massage (although this may seem like the very hardest thing to try, being taught this as a skill with a specific routine and a focus on the baby's response rather than necessarily the feel of it, can actually make this more possible to do for some)

What would help you to increase your physical contact with your baby?

____

____

____

____

____

____

Bringing this to ourselves too

We can again learn from our baby in terms of creating the foundations of our compassionate mind towards ourselves. We never grow out of needing physical closeness and warmth (physical and/or psychological warmth) as they are powerful regulators of our emotions and physical state (indeed it is thought that an early function of oxytocin was to bring a parent and their offspring close for thermoregulation). These remain an important part of our soothing/safeness system. Like our baby, we will have individual differences in the degree of physical closeness and warmth that feels 'just right' to us, and this will be dependent upon our personality, neurological make-up such as autism, factors in the moment such as tiredness, annoyance, hormonal cycle, and so on.

In terms of physical closeness, touch, and emotional and physical warmth – what has helped you to feel settled and soothed over the past few days?

(It might be people, pets, sitting under a soft weighted blanket, holding a warm drink, holding a heavy cup of coffee, sitting in the sun, putting your socks on, putting a big jumper on, sitting on the sofa squidging into some big cushions, cuddling your baby, a warm bath, a hug, a hand on your arm, a warm smile, or warm words to you.)

____

____

____

____

____

Bring to mind your compassionate self or compassionate other – what aspects of physical and emotional closeness, touch and warmth do they bring to you?

____

____

____

____

____

2) Taking the pressure off

When we are trying hard to get things right, especially when they are important to us, or when our critic takes hold of what we are struggling with, then we can move into our threat system. When it comes to synchrony and mind-mindedness, as we have seen, we need to be in the soothing/safeness system rather than the threat system. So it might be that taking the pressure off ourselves and bringing our compassionate mind to our efforts, allows us to start moving into our safeness/soothing system where mind-mindedness and synchrony are now assisted rather than hindered.

There are some wonderful teaching programmes that help parents who for one reason or another are struggling to interact with their baby. It can be very helpful to have a clear programme to follow which provides the 'scaffolding' around how to be with our baby. This can be particularly helpful if we feel at a loss to know how to be with and interact with them.

One such programme is called 'Watch, Wait and Wonder'. These three words really sum up the whole pattern, in body and mind, that we use in mindfulness. It also sums up the pattern in our baby when they are introduced to something new and interesting. Just imagining being with your baby in this way can take away the pressure to be singing songs you might not know, or playing games that you cannot think of or were never shown. Instead, what your baby is wired to want from you is your warm, interested and delighted attention. Just watching what they are doing ('Watch'), giving space to wait for their 'initiatives' – their movements, facial expressions and sounds ('Wait'), and for you to receive them like catching a ball that they have thrown to you. But not just catching it blankly, receiving it with wonder, delight, joy and warm interest ('Wonder').

'Wonder' of course is sadly very hard to experience when we have pre- or postnatal depression, but it can be possible if the depression is not too severe. Even the tiniest flicker of wonder and warmth in us, or the intention to be interested and warm, will be registered by our baby. In fact, the work using videos of interactions between mums and their baby on Mother and Baby units shows that even when mothers are very depressed or poorly, they still connect and respond to their baby, albeit with less energy and 'fizz'.

Sadly, their depression means that they believe they don't. Video interaction work is a very powerful tool to help parents to see with their own eyes the tiny but powerful dance and interaction that they have with their baby, even when they are feeling very depressed and believe with certainty that they are not responding positively at all. It also helps them to see what they are doing that is so powerful for the baby; a baby is born able to detect these tiny moments – they don't need big demonstrations of enthusiasm. Seeing what they have done, that the baby is responding to them, provides a map of what to do more of. The technique allows us to be our own teachers. It also teaches us this kind of attention – drawing our mind to what is going well, rather than what is going wrong – which is what our mind tends to do if left to its own devices, particularly when it is feeling down or anxious, or in other words, under threat. The video work also provides a record of interactions that they might have been too poorly to remember.

Another approach which can be viewed for free on the internet is 'Watch Me Play', which is very similar, with the same philosophy of following the baby with a calm, interested, curious mind.

These, and other similar interventions, are becoming available in more and more areas, so do ask your health visitor or GP if there are any that you could attend.

It also doesn't need to be just on the mother, who might find that the pressure of this is an additional burden on top of all she is already struggling with, meaning she gets even further away from feeling delight and warmth. Remember, our brains have been set up in the context of living in groups where there would be many people delighted in the birth of our baby, who are not exhausted, anxious or depressed. Our baby would be experiencing many of these interactions, allowing the mother to be looked after, to rest and to recuperate. The responsibility for our baby, who is a welcomed and precious member of 'the village', would be held by many, not just the mother or even just the parent. The saying 'It takes a village to raise a child' is such an important one to hold in mind.

What would help you to take the pressure off with regard to your baby? (Remember to use your compassionate mind rather than threat mind to help you answer this.) Who might help you with this? What would you advise your baby if they were fully grown and had become a parent and had come to you with this worry?

___

___

___

___

___

Reflections and notes: What would you like to take hold of and remember from this section about priming mind-mindedness and synchrony through proximity and touch and through taking the pressure off? What would you like to take forward and try? What might be your next steps?

____

____

____

____

____

Module 33: The compassionate mind, mind-mindedness, synchrony and attachment: Bringing it all together

An example of what the mind-minded, synchronous, compassionate mind might look like in action

(Remember, this is hard to do if we are suffering from depression, have little support, feel exhausted and so on – the intention here is not to make us feel like a failure, but to know what a mind-minded, synchronous, compassionate mind might look like in relation to parenting, so we can see when we are doing this, and have a guide to where we are trying to get to as well):

This scenario is of two parents who have taken their baby out for lunch at a café and have just arrived there. These are examples of interactions with the baby:

- Explaining to the baby what is going to happen – 'We are going to get some lunch. Let's find a table – here we are. Shall we see if there is a highchair for you?'
- Giving a familiar preparation before lifting the baby up into the highchair – 'Ooh, Up. Here we go.'
- Gently putting in the highchair.
- Giving a toy immediately – anticipating their mind that they won't want to be in the highchair.
- Giving them their water first before looking at the menu yourselves.
- Giving a snack as know that waiting will be hard for them, especially if hungry.
- Responding to initiatives – in a particular way – with a delighted face, welcoming their communications and 'conversation'.
- Talking to them about their surroundings – what they can see.
- Monitoring their state and responding to it.
- Anticipating what might happen when you go to the toilet and leave them with their other parent. Helping them with this if they might find it hard.
- Keep bringing face-to-face contact with them, avoiding time looking at phone, and including them or acknowledging them when talking to others.
- Notice how you give them food that shows you understand their mind, e.g. breaking it into pieces that fit their hands, helping them with it, putting it on a spoon which they then hold, etc.

- Dealing with refusal of food calmly and with acknowledgement of what they are communicating, e.g. that is enough of that food, or enough of that food at the moment.
- Preparing them that you are going to wipe their face, doing it gently, and then signalling you have finished, or helping them to wipe own face if old enough.
- Taking out of highchair with care. Checking they are steady when putting them down.
- Explaining what is coming next – 'Shall we go and see all the stones?'

Your reflections on this. What would you like to take note of and remember?

____

____

____

____

____

Exercise: Me at my imaginary compassionate best with my baby

When we imagine something 'at its best' it allows us to make conscious just what this looks like for us. It then makes it much easier, and much more likely, that we will move closer toward making it a reality.

First get into your compassionate mind:

- Sit back in your chair, with your feet flat on the ground hip width apart.
- Feel the ground underneath your feet.
- Sit upright 'like a mountain' or mighty oak tree with your dignified posture. Bring your shoulders up to your ears then drop them down and back, feeling the space in your chest.
- Close your eyes or allow your gaze to rest lightly on an object.
- Bring your warm, kind face and your warm, kind voice tone to your breath. Perhaps greeting it as if you are really pleased to have come across it, 'Hello breath!'
- Allow your in breath to slow down and move deep into the base of your lungs, notice the pause,

and then allow your out breath to become really slow, gentle and smooth. Perhaps use your 'ocean breathing' where you make the sound of the sea by breathing out through your mouth with your throat constricted. You are aiming for a sound you'd make if you were trying to 'fog' a mirror or pair of glasses for cleaning. This slows down and extends the out breath even more.

- Move into that part of yourself that tries to be as helpful as it can, that has great wisdom and strength, courage and warmth. From this place, see what flows when you answer these questions:

How would the 'You at your compassionate best' be with your baby when they first wake up in the morning?

What might your day look like with your baby?

How would you feed your baby?

What might you do with your baby during the day?

How would you be with your baby?

How would you be with yourself?

What might bedtime look like for you and your baby?

What might dealing with a long bout of crying look like? (Remember the oxygen mask principle; compassion to self first.)

What might responding to your baby's repeated waking at night look like?

Reflections: What was it like for you to do this exercise?

____

____

____

____

____

What would you like to take from this to hold onto and remember?

____

____

____

____

____

Practice: Bringing together secure base, safe haven, mind-mindedness and synchrony into our compassionate other/image

- Make yourself comfortable, sitting with your feet on the floor, hip width apart, eyes closed or gently focused on an object. Slow down your in and your out breath, breathing slow, deep and smooth, and bring a warm, kind face and voice to yourself.
- Now imagine that a person or being arrives who embodies all the aspects of this section. They are a secure attachment figure who provides you with a secure base and a safe haven. You know that you could lean into them, depend on them, be helped and encouraged by them, and settled by them if needed. They know your mind well and are responsive and attuned to you. Imagine being met now by a person or being who is here just for you. They have a deep wish to help you and to bring joy into your life.

- You are aware of this being's warmth and kindness. It seems to be deeply connected to you and seems to experience real joy in just being here with you. It knows you inside and out. There is nothing you need to explain to it or be worried about it finding out. It understands your history, your human tricky brain set-up that we all have, your genes that you didn't choose but which influence you, and has seen all the way back into previous generations of your family, so it knows just what you struggle with and what you need. It tunes in to how you are feeling and is working out what you might need or want right now. You might want company, to talk something through, to do something enjoyable together, to be light-hearted together, or just to carry on with what you are doing, knowing there is someone who has got your back as soon as you need it.
- Your compassionate being or other comes as close or as far as you need, just monitoring your body, what you say, your expressions, in order to work out what seems just right to you. Perhaps you need it to sit with you, just put a gentle hand on your back occasionally when it senses you need to know it's still here. Perhaps you need it to sit close or to hug you, or perhaps you are happy for it to be seated, busy doing something at the side of the room, or just in another room so you can easily call it when you need to.
- No matter how you are feeling, or how you react to it, it understands and accepts that. It will be concerned and moved if you are struggling, even if you get angry at it, collapse into tears, or ignore it completely even when it tries to help.
- You sense its heartfelt wish for you. Notice how it feels in your body to take this in – that it wishes this for you.
- You feel totally safe in its presence. It is steady, strong and withstands whatever you throw at it. You understand that because this is your compassionate being, it will be with you for your whole life. It will never leave you. Notice how it feels to take this in.
- When you interact with it, it matches your emotions; when you are joyful, it is joyful too. When you are angry, it acknowledges how strong this is and gives you the understanding and the space that you need in this moment. When you are quiet, it is quiet too.

- You sense that it is really trying to monitor your mind and adjust what it anticipates you need next accordingly. Being with it makes you feel at ease. There is an easy flow to your interactions, like a rather beautiful dance that would bring you joy if you were to watch it. You feel settled and calm, knowing you have this being in your life. It makes you feel stronger and more courageous, knowing that, with it, you can go out and try new things, difficult things, things that will help you in the long run or bring you joy, and that it will help you, encourage you, and be there for you if it is harder than you thought, or all goes wrong.
- Having it here with you, allows you to know that it will help you when things get difficult with your baby. You notice you can think more clearly about what will be helpful for you and your baby. That you feel steadier and stronger and that you can be more at ease with yourself and your baby.
- You also become aware that it takes great joy seeing you with your baby and is moved and proud when you work at the struggles of motherhood. Notice how it feels to have this being taking such joy and delight in you and your baby, even when things get tough. You sense it is just happy to be able to be part of your life.
- Stay here as long as you wish.
- When you are ready, take hold of your sense of this compassionate being. Perhaps imagine taking a picture of it, or give it a name, or focus in on a particular part of it that sums it up for you, so that you can more easily bring it to mind when you need to. Perhaps you can choose an object or picture or write some words that will bring this being to mind another time, particularly when you are struggling.
- Bring your attention to the sounds in your room, allowing them to flow in through your ears. Shift your attention to the feel of your feet in contact with the floor and your hands on your lap, perhaps moving them. Notice the feel of the chair underneath you, supporting you. When you are ready, gently open your eyes.
- See if you can move off into the next part of your day, just holding on to the sense of this compassionate presence.

End of practice.

What was this practice like for you?

____

____

____

____

____

What would you like to remember and take forward from this practice?

____

____

____

____

____

To summarise this section:

1. Begins with compassionate mind – intention, wish, to do the best we can in helping us and our baby interact in this sensitive, synchronous way – commitment to work on this, courage to try this, wisdom to understand this is important – do the practice of compassionate self/compassionate other, embodying both the steadiness and the flexibility.

⇩

2. Then physical proximity and warm, calm, positive interactions – creating flow of oxytocin in mother and baby

⇩

3. Enables mentalisation so can really tune in to what the baby is 'telling' us, i.e. positive affect and interactions that encourage us keep it going. A sense of 'that is great, do more

of that' from our baby. And the sense of 'that's enough', or 'I didn't quite like that' that our baby's affect and behaviour tells us so we change what we are doing.

⇩

4. Which enables synchrony – the moment-to-moment 'dance' of interactions.

⇩

5. Which builds brain, oxytocin and heart synchrony.

⇩

6. Which provides the foundation of the secure base with us, and of the ability to self-regulate and interact with others.

⇩

7. Which builds more sophisticated synchrony.

⇩

8. Which builds more sophisticated self-regulatory and interactive abilities. (A positive 'snowball' which grows and grows throughout life.)

⇩

9. This spreads out across all other interactions enabling the ability to engage in all three flows of compassion: compassion to others, compassion from others, compassion to ourselves.

Reflections and notes: What would you like to take hold of and remember from this section about bringing together the compassionate mind, mind-mindedness, synchrony and attachment? What would you like to take forward and try? What might be your next steps?

____

____

____

____

____

Section 6:

Bringing our compassionate mind to the complexities of ourselves

Module 34: Our different selves (multiple selves)

When something happens to us, people might ask, 'So how did you feel about that?' or, 'What did you think about that?', with the implication that we only have one response. However, we often have more than one response. And we can have contrasting responses that cause us to want to do opposite things at the same time, such as to retreat but also lash out, or to be angry and also to cry. These might make us feel overwhelmed or like our brain can't think clearly. Yet if we spend some time with all the different parts that contribute to this state of 'overwhelmed' it can become clearer and make sense. Sometimes our strongest (or apparently only) reaction might mask an emotion that more accurately represents how we feel but is scarier for us to experience.

Our different emotions can affect many aspects of us and act like mini 'selves'. It can be very enlightening and helpful to see just what happens when a particular 'self' or pattern takes hold of us.

What follows is an exercise usually referred to as 'multiple selves'. It is one that can offer an immense amount in terms of how we understand ourselves, our baby and others. It is well worth having a go with, and the language of different selves or parts will be referred to throughout the rest of this book.

Exercise: Multiple selves

(See https://overcoming.co.uk/715/resources-to-download for downloadable 'multiple selves' forms)

Step One:

Firstly, pick an issue that you want to explore from the different parts of you. For this exercise we will use the experience of imagining that you have had an argument with somebody that you care about.

Take an A4 piece of paper and fold it in half one way and then the other way. Open it back up. The creases should make a cross shape. At the point where all the lines cross write a word that summarises what you are going to be thinking about. In this case write 'argument'.

Step Two:

In the bottom left-hand rectangle, we are going to start with 'angry self' so write that as a heading. Now get into that angry part of you as if you are stepping into its shoes and body:

1. **What thoughts is your angry self having about this argument?** (Write them as if you are saying or shouting them out loud to the other person.)

2. **What are you feeling in your body? (e.g. heart rate, breathing rate, tension, etc.) Where are you feeling it in the angry part of your body?**

3. **If these feelings were to grow and grow, what would be the urge in your body? What would your body want to do if you let it?**

4. Where is your attention focused?

5. What images are popping into your mind? (These might be cartoon-like/pictures/a sense of how you imagine yourself from the outside, e.g. like a volcano erupting, like a cartoon figure jumping up and down with steam coming out of its ears.)

6. What kinds of memories come up? How far back do these memories go?

7. What does the angry self really need for it to settle?

Step Three:

Now step out of your 'angry self'. It can go off and have a cup of tea. And then step into your 'anxious self'. Write your responses in the bottom right-hand rectangle.

1. What does your anxious self think about this argument? What thoughts are running through your anxious self's head?

2. What is happening in your anxious self's body? How do you know that you are feeling anxious?

3. If these feelings and sensations were to grow and grow, what would be the urge in your anxious self's body? What would your body want to do if you let it?

4. Where is your anxious self's attention focused?

5. What images pop into your anxious self's mind? (These might be cartoon images, pictures or fantasies of what your anxious self might look like from the outside, e.g. looking very small, or wide eyed 'like a frightened rabbit'.)

6. What memories are coming up? How far back do these memories go?

7. What does your anxious self really need in order for it to settle?

Step Four:

Step out of your anxious self, like you are taking off a set of clothes, and step into your 'sad self'. Your anxious self can go off and get a cup of tea. Write your responses in the top right-hand rectangle.

1. What are your sad self's thoughts about this argument?

2. What is happening in your sad self's body? How does it know that it is feeling sad?

____

____

____

____

____

3. If these feelings and body sensations were to grow and grow, what would be the urge in your sad self's body? What would your sad self do if you let it?

____

____

____

____

____

4. Where is your sad self's attention focused?

____

____

____

____

____

5. What images pop into your sad self's mind?

____

6. What type of memories are coming up for your sad self? How far back might these memories go?

7. What does the sad self really need for it to settle?

Step Five:

Step out of your sad self – it can go off and have a cup of tea with your angry self and anxious self.

Step Six:

Imagining your angry, anxious and sad selves sat in a café together having a cup of tea:

How might your angry self feel about your anxious self?

How might your angry self feel about your sad self?

How might your anxious self feel about your angry self?

How might your anxious self feel about your sad self?

How might your sad self feel about your angry self?

How might your sad self feel about your anxious self?

Step Seven:

Now, like we did with the other selves, we are going to step into our compassionate self.

But to do this, we need to do our 'compassionate self' practice first:

- So, sit supported by your chair, feet flat on the floor hip width apart in your 'dignified' posture ('body like a mountain'), bringing your shoulders up to your ears, and dropping them back and down. Close your eyes or soften your gaze.
- Bring your warm, kind voice and face to yourself and your breath, perhaps in your mind greeting yourself and your breath as if you are really pleased to have come across them.
- Slow down your in breath, bringing it deeply and smoothly into the base of your lungs, and really slow down your out breath, using your ocean breathing (making the noise of the ocean in the back of your throat) or toning (deep hum) on each out breath. Feel your body slowing down with each out breath. You might notice it increasing in its feeling of steadiness and stability.
- Now move into that part of you that wishes to be as caring and helpful as it can. The part that can be courageous and has great strength, perhaps even surprisingly so. The part of you that has gathered such wisdom over your lifetime; that understands that human minds have been shaped by evolution, by genes, by experiences. That we are wired to want to avoid threat and seek safeness. That we have a whole set of emotions and behaviours that we didn't choose.
- Imagine now looking at this argument from this place of compassion, this place of wisdom and strength, steadiness and calm, warmth and kindness.

1. What thoughts are coming into your mind about this argument, from the point of view of your compassionate self? Write your responses in the top left rectangle.

____

____

____

____

____

2. What are you feeling in your compassionate self's body? Where are you feeling these sensations in your body?

____

____

____

3. **If these feelings were to grow and grow, what would be the urge in your body? What would your body like to do if you let it?**

4. **Where is your attention focused?**

5. **What images pop into your mind?**

6. **What memories come up?**

____

____

____

____

____

How does your compassionate mind feel about your:

Angry self?

____

____

____

Anxious self?

____

____

____

Sad self?

____

____

____

1. Compassionate self:	3. Sad self:
i. Thoughts ii. Body iii. Urges iv. Attention v. Images vi. Memories	i. Thoughts ii. Body iii. Urges iv. Attention v. Images vi. Memories vii. Settle
2. Angry self:	**4. Anxious self:**
i. Thoughts ii. Body iii. Urges iv. Attention v. Images vi. Memories vii. Settle	i. Thoughts ii. Body iii. Urges iv. Attention v. Images vi. Memories vii. Settle

Reflections on this multiple-selves exercise: What were some of the aspects that you particularly noticed? What are some of the things you would like to remember from this exercise?

____

____

____

____

____

Take-away points from multiple selves

There are so many learning points from this exercise. Hopefully, these include a concept that becomes a key part of understanding yourself, your baby and others. Here are just a few of the take-away points that people have discovered in doing the multiple selves:

Each part acts as an entire 'self'.	The angry part thinks angry thoughts, has a particular pattern in the body (e.g. fast heart rate, clenched teeth/fists), angry images, angry urges (e.g. shout, punch, kick, push), attention focused outwards, angry memories. These are all different to those of the anxious self and the sad self. So, the pattern or 'self' we are in takes us over entirely.
If we want to think, or behave, etc., in a different way then we need to swap systems/patterns/selves/parts.	We may try to think compassionately or wish others were kinder, yet our circumstances are pushing us into our threat system. This is not our fault. To think differently we need to switch systems, by changing environments perhaps, or by consciously doing practices such as compassionate self.
The threat mind can only come up with threat solutions.	The threat mind will struggle to ever find reassurance as it is designed to always respond with 'yes, but . . . ' and see the worst case. To find a solution we need to switch out of threat mind and into the compassionate mind.

The threat mind only pulls up threat memories.	We cannot even remember better or more helpful things as that is not what the threat mind is designed to remember. We need to switch systems from threat to soothing/safeness to be able to access memories, such as people that could help us, things we can do, rather than threat memories of being alone, and things we can't do, etc.
Each self will feel like the truth and a fact.	When a part of us has got hold of us, it feels like it is our true self and its memories, thoughts, etc., are true facts. In fact, all of these change like a weather pattern. We move in and out of our selves or patterns all the time. But we can choose which is most helpful to us and learn how to swap selves (although this isn't easy).
Even the wish or decision to switch systems will be governed by the one we are in.	So, even if we recognise that we are in one self or pattern that is not helping us, e.g. the demotivated self, and want to switch systems into, say, the compassionate self, then the demotivated self may well say 'well, what's the point in doing the compassionate self? How is a couple of minutes' exercise going to help anything when our life is terrible?' The demotivated self *would* say that as that is how it is designed to respond, so it's important to have faith that giving the compassionate self a go may help you to move into a different physical and psychological state that gives you access to totally different memories, solutions and so on. Even if your threat system tells you otherwise.
Each pattern or self can react to another one.	If we are feeling angry, for example, then the anxious part of us may get scared or sad, so we can end up with multiple parts of us all activated at once.

Opposing motives or actions of different selves can make us feel overwhelmed or like our brain has 'blown a fuse'.	We may feel both the urge to attack and defend, and also the urge to run away or cry. This can lead to unclear and confusing feelings, and we can become immobilised and unable to take action. Once we unpick each separate self, it all usually becomes much clearer and more understandable. Our compassionate self can then help us find a way forward.
A part or self can be linked or conditioned to another part.	For example, children are born with the capacity to be angry and frustrated. If a parent gets angry at them for being angry, then anger gets connected to a feeling of anxiety and/or shame. Eventually when the child (or adult) feels a little spark of anger, then anxiety and shame may come up as well, and may well become the more dominant emotion. In the end it may be hard to detect any anger in ourselves at all.
Particular emotions may seem to disappear from our repertoire.	We might say we never get angry or never get sad, for example. (However, like our baby, we are born with all the emotions.) This may be because we learned that to be angry or to be sad led to a significant person in our lives getting angrier or abandoning us (physically or psychologically) or getting upset. We learned that having the emotion was not helpful or was actually harmful to us because of its consequences. But actually we need to be able to access all of our emotions so they can guide our compassionate mind as to what we are struggling with and need.
Usually, people can order the different selves into a list from 'easiest' to 'hardest'.	This can be enlightening. The easiest emotions may be the ones we feel safest to have and the hardest may be the ones that we might really need in our lives but struggle to express or manage.

Each threat self wants the same thing in order for it to settle.	Usually each threat self is after the same thing; to be heard, to be understood, to be accepted, to be safe. The compassionate self is already by its very nature in a settled state where its motivation is to listen, try to understand, accept, be helpful; all of which is what each threat self is ultimately seeking.
The compassionate self is a very different system to the others.	Because it comes from the safeness/soothing system, it uses different physiological and brain systems. So, its attention is broad compared to the narrow, focused threat system selves – it attends to not just one or other person involved in the argument, but both. It looks even wider than that too, understanding the circumstances and influences that have created both people and that this isn't their fault. It looks to the future too and puts this argument into perspective and context.
The compassionate self accepts and integrates all the other selves.	Whereas each threat part reacts with threat to the other parts, the compassionate self understands, accepts and offers help to the threat parts. Also, the part of the brain that generates the compassionate mind has the ability to integrate or bring together different aspects into one whole picture. Whereas the brain area responsible for threat separates things into categories and black and white thinking, etc. So, rather than believing 'I am an angry person', or 'I am a rubbish mother', the compassionate mind helps us to understand that, like every human, we are made up of *all* those bits – sometimes we are angry, sometimes we are a bit rubbish and might want to make amends and try to do it a bit better next time, sometimes we are helpful, sometimes we are courageous, and so on . . .

The final step of switching to the compassionate self is then turning back to any threat selves.	When we move pattern from, say, the angry self into the compassionate self, it can feel like the angry self has just been abandoned. However, the final part of the process is that, once we are in our compassionate mind, we then turn to the angry, anxious or sad self, but from this position of strength, wisdom and caring. The compassionate part listens to what the threat part has to say and tries to help it as best it can.
We can switch quickly between each threat self, but the compassionate self takes time and practice to get into.	You might have noticed that we were swapping in and out of the threat selves very quickly, but for the compassionate self we did a practice. This is because the threat system is a fast-acting system. It is always revved and ready to go just in case we need it. It can take quite a bit of work to swap out of threat and into the safeness/soothing system. So, it is understandable that responding from a place of compassion is not easy, even for the most practised, especially when we are having to move out of threat first. Being able to approach things from our compassionate mind is a constant process of falling into threat, noticing that we have, getting out, and getting into compassion, falling into threat again . . . That's why strength and commitment are so important – to allow us to keep pointing ourselves back in the right direction, all the way through our lives.

Troubleshooting multiple selves

When I am trying to stay in one self, I end up in another one.	Notice which emotion or self seems linked to another one. There may be a reason why one emotion tends to pull up another one, so stay curious about this. These may have become linked due to experiences earlier in your life. If possible, return and give voice to the original emotion – it may well have some wisdom or insight to offer. If it feels hard to stay there, imagine 'if', e.g. 'I know you find it hard to be angry, but *if* someone were to be angry about this, what might they say/think/feel in their body?', etc.
I get stuck in one self.	Often there is a self which is easier to be in, or that we are quite enjoying letting have its say, or that we are getting too immersed in. It is important to hear from all parts of us. So, we can check with the part we feel stuck in: 'Anything else you need me to hear? I can always come back to you if there is more.' And then imagine stepping out of it, letting it leave the room to go and have a cup of tea, and then imagine stepping into the next one. It can help to swap chairs or move your chair to more clearly separate the parts.

Multiple selves in action: Some examples

Note: Only angry, anxious and sad selves are picked for these exercises. Many other parts may show up, e.g. jealous part, disgusted part, etc., so just add any other parts that may be showing up for you.

- **WHEN YOUR BABY REPEATEDLY WAKES IN THE NIGHT:**

How are your angry, anxious and sad selves responding to this?

____

____

____

____

Step into your compassionate mind, or imagine having your compassionate image with you – how would this part understand your angry, anxious and sad parts?

____

____

____

____

How might your compassionate mind be with these other parts? How might it try to help them?

____

____

____

____

What parts/selves might be coming up for your baby when they wake in the night?

How might your compassionate mind be with, and help, these parts of your baby?

How might you go to your baby the next time they wake when you have your compassionate mind with you?

- **WHEN A RELATIVE OFFERS 'HELPFUL' ADVICE:**

How are your angry, anxious and sad selves responding to this?

How would your compassionate self be with your angry, anxious and sad selves?

How might the angry, anxious and sad selves of your relative be influencing their decision to give you this advice?

How might your compassionate self help you with this situation?

How might your compassionate self help you and your relative with this situation?

- **WHEN YOUR PARTNER IS TETCHY AND IRRITABLE:**

How might your angry, anxious and sad selves be reacting to this?

How might your compassionate mind/image be with these different parts of you?

What might your partner's angry, anxious and sad selves have to say?

How might your compassionate mind/image be with your partner's different selves?

How might your compassionate mind/image be with both you and your partner?

- **WHEN YOU FEEL REGRET AT HAVING A BABY:**

How might your angry, anxious and sad selves be responding to having had a baby?

How might your compassionate mind be with each of these selves?

How might your compassionate mind/image be with you? How might it help you?

Reflections and notes: What would you like to take hold of and remember from this section about our multiple selves? What would you like to take forward and try? What might be your next steps?

Module 35: Formulation

Hopefully, a kind of story is coming together for you as you read this book. The formulation is about bringing in the finer detail of your own story, into the more general story we have of us as humans and as mothers; that as humans we appear in this world, without choosing to. We arrive with a brain, body, emotions, genes, etc., that we didn't choose but that can be quite tricky for us to work out and navigate. We are wired to want to attach to others, to feel safe and to be able to operate at our best when we do feel safe. And, for humans, a significant source of safeness is being held positively in the minds of other people. We are social beings.

On top of this, we have the impact of brain changes that occur during and after pregnancy, which we did not choose either, but which will shape us profoundly too.

We also have upbringings and experiences, particularly those early in life, which shape our brains and our strategies (conscious or unconscious) to get through life with as little threat and suffering as possible, and which even shape how our genes play out. We don't choose these either. If we were brought up in a different family, such as our neighbours to the left of us or a family in a different country, we might have been very different to the version of ourselves that we are today. This is not our fault, but it gives us our particular shape and story.

But we also know that humans are adaptable and that our brains continue to wire up and respond to our environment until we die. So, we can also take hold of our destiny or story and have some influence over how we would like it to unfold from here. We can help ourselves become a slightly different version to the one we currently are if we wish. This book is all about helping us to use compassion to shape the version of ourselves in a way that science has found to be particularly helpful, literally by training and changing our brain.

We can begin to take steps that take us down a different path, and although at the beginning we aren't far from our original path, over time we can end up in a very different place. This book helps us to begin, or to carry on that journey.

Some of what makes us us

- Our brain and body, including a set of emotions and behaviours shaped for us by evolution
- Our genetics and epigenetics
- Our upbringing and experiences
- The environment we are currently living in and the people around us
- Our brain and body that has been changed by pregnancy and child-rearing
- Our baby and the interactions between us and them (these interactions affect our brain and body)

One way of working out what has made us the way we are, but that also gives us the start of a roadmap as to where we go next, is by something called a formulation.

The formulation used in the compassionate mind approach is a table with just four columns. Although it looks simple, it can become as detailed as you wish. Even if you don't fill this out for yourself, the concepts it teaches can be very powerful and helpful.

The **background** column might include significant experiences you have had or are still having with regard to your immediate family, extended family, friends, neighbours or school. It might also include things like losses, health issues for yourself or others, moving house or school.

The **fear** column is about the worries, concerns and fears that arose as a consequence of those experiences listed in 'background'. These fears are split into external fears, which are fears we develop about other people, and internal fears, which are fears we develop about ourselves.

As humans we have evolved to stay safe and to avoid threat, so we develop **safety strategies** to try to ensure, as best as possible, that these fears don't come true again. These safety strategies might be unconscious. For example, as a baby we might learn that if we turn away from our mother when she is a bit too overwhelming when she plays with us, she gets cross and goes away from us. We learn to keep looking at her even when we feel overwhelmed because we need our mother close by for survival. This isn't something we have consciously decided to do, it has just been automatically conditioned into us through biological processes that we are not aware of. A conscious safety strategy, on the other hand, might be one where we tell ourselves 'I keep getting hurt in relationships, so I am not going to get involved with anyone ever again'. It is a decision that we are aware we have made.

Although the intention behind a safety strategy is to keep us safe, sometimes they can have downsides or **unintended consequences**. So, in the examples above, the child that unconsciously overrides their biological need to dip out of an overwhelming interaction in order to regulate, may find that as they grow up, they never really get to know their own needs and will always be focused outwards on others. They end up getting exhausted, overwhelmed and resentful without perhaps understanding why. The person who decides never to have any more relationships to avoid getting hurt may end up being alone.

At the bottom of the unintended consequences column is a section that says 'self-to-self relating'. This is how we feel about and relate to ourselves when these unintended consequences happen. So, the person that attends to the needs of others and not themselves may then feel like they might explode with anger or implode with overwhelm. They may say to themselves something like, 'You are so dramatic. No-one wants to be with a needy drama queen.' They are now flipped back into the fear that their needs will make people turn away and abandon them again.

The person who ends up alone may criticise themselves for having no-one – 'See, you are unlovable'.

When we relate to ourselves in a critical or threat-based way, we trigger our fears, which trigger our safety strategies, resulting in unintended consequences – and so it goes round with us getting stuck in these loops.

Figure 5: An example formulation

Background	Fears		Safety strategies	Unintended consequences
Key events in your life, particularly relationships	What fears or worries your experiences gave you about others (external fears) or yourself (internal fears)		Conscious or unconscious ways of making sure these fears didn't happen again	The downsides of these safety strategies
	External fears ('Others are . . . ')	**Internal fears** (' I am . . . ')		
Older sister was 'a handful' – she had some kind of behavioural/ psychiatric disorder and could be violent and unpredictable	*Scary, demanding, selfish, destructive, horrible*	*Critical, horrible, judgemental, jealous, scared, sad, lonely, angry, resentful*	*Be nice to her so she doesn't attack me* *Keep rage and jealousy down by criticising myself and keeping people at a distance*	*Feel a fake, that people will discover I am not very nice really so I criticise myself and keep people at a distance – end up feeling alone* *Feel really strong emotions, such as rage and resentment to my baby when they are 'a handful', which seem to erupt out of nowhere and scare me*
Mother anxious and short-tempered	*Angry, scared, unable to protect me, weak*	*Contemptuous, angry, sad, alone, scared*	*Try to appease people, be 'the good one'* *Be independent. Don't rely on others, only self*	*Don't get my needs met.* *Feel resentful* *Don't get the help from others that I need, particularly now I have a baby, so feel exhausted, resentful, scared to ask for help*

Dad away a lot	*Absent. Not there when you need them* *More important than me*	*Sad, unprotected, abandoned, hurt,* *unloved, unlovable,* *uninteresting, unimportant, angry, resentful, jealous*	*Try not to put too much on partner in case they start working away more to get away from me*	*Feel alone, unprotected, abandoned, unloved – the very thing I fear* *Don't ask for the help I need so feel exhausted and resentful* *Baby doesn't get to spend the time they need with partner*
I tried to care for and protect younger brother because my mother was an alcoholic	*Needy, helpless, vulnerable* *Burdensome* *Embarrassing* *Shameful* *Unavailable* *Unpredictable* *'Pathetic'*	*Overwhelmed* *Out of my depth* *Resentful, I am more grown up and capable than my mum* *Contemptuous of her*	*Be 'the grown up responsible one'*	*Become the one that others lean on but then can't be the one who leans on them now I have my baby* *I wouldn't know who I was if I was the one who needed help, and I would look down on myself, so I must keep struggling on. But feel scared it will all crumble and I will no longer be able to cope at all*
				Self-to-self relating (How we relate to ourselves can loop us back to our internal and external fears) *If people really knew me, they would see that I am not nice and kind but actually angry and resentful, even of my baby. If they found out they would abandon me and I would end up alone, which is awful for anyone, but much harder when I've had a baby and really need help. I am horrible, a failure, a mess.*

My formulation

Background	Fears		Safety strategies	Unintended consequences
(Key events in your life, particularly relationships)	(What fears or worries your experiences gave you about others (external fears) or yourself (internal fears)		(Conscious or unconscious ways of making sure these fears didn't happen again)	(The downsides of these safety strategies)
	External fears (Others are . . .)	**Internal fears** (I am . . .)		

				Self-to-self relating (How I feel about myself when these unintended consequences happen – these often leave me feeling the very thing I fear, which then sets off my safety strategies and then the unintended consequences get caught in a loop)

There is space in the back of the book for you to complete your own formulation for easier reference in the future. Alternatively write this in your own journal or download the sheets from https://overcoming.co.uk/715/resources-to-download.

Tips for writing out your formulation

Draw the four columns on a rough sheet of paper. This might help to make it easier to just jot down what comes to mind in the column you think it goes in rather than feel under pressure to get it right. It doesn't matter if you are not sure. You can then move things around, cross things out, draw arrows, whatever you like.

It can be easier to start writing out your background as a kind of timeline, jotting down what jumps out at you as important. You don't need to analyse why, just trust that it has jumped out at you for a reason. This reason may become clear as you work through the formulation (or it may become clear later in life, or perhaps never. Just trust that for whatever reason this feels important to you).

You might then begin filling the columns across from each event.

Sometimes people prefer to think about one key memory and use the columns to analyse this in detail.

You don't have to work from left to right across the columns. You may think of something that is an issue for you, for example, and then wonder about which column it might fit best in. Then work out the other columns in relation to that. For example, a person in one of our groups realised that she always kept friends at arm's length and panicked when someone from the group asked her round for coffee. She wanted to formulate this and so we drew out the four columns. She decided that this was probably a safety strategy. (One way of checking whether or not it is a safety strategy is to imagine that for some reason you could no longer do this safety strategy. Then see what that might be like. If a fear arises, then it is probably a safety strategy. It can also reveal the fear, which then goes in the 'fear' column.)

She then wondered what the fear might be that this safety strategy protected her from. She thought it was probably because she felt like she wasn't a very nice person really and that if this person got close, they would discover this. She then wondered where this fear that she wasn't a very nice person came from and realised that her mother had been quite critical and attacking of her. This left her feeling 'bad' inside. It was this 'bad' feeling that she was worried would be discovered by others.

She then looked at the unintended consequence of keeping people at arm's length and found that she always felt lonely and an outsider, never connected or properly part of a group. She then criticised herself for this, which then made her feel the same 'bad' that her mother did. So, you can really start anywhere with the formulation.

Working with one particular memory can be exceedingly helpful and eye-opening. Choose a memory that keeps popping up for you. Check you feel OK to spend time with it. (It might be one for another time or for exploring with someone you feel comfortable with.) This will go in the 'background' column but for now just write it in the middle of a piece of paper. Put a circle around it. Now on the right-hand side of the paper write all the things that you felt during that event. Go through each 'self' as we did in 'multiple selves' – angry self, anxious self, sad self. Any other selves? Are there any feelings that you find it hard to feel, or that you would feel if somebody you cared about was in that situation? What might have happened in that moment if you had shown that emotion? How might the other person, or key people in your life, have reacted if you had shown it? These answers can give insights into emotions in ourselves that we might be scared to have. These would then go in the 'internal fears' column.

On the left-hand side of the circle right down all the things that you noticed about the other person in relation to yourself in this memory. For example, you might write, 'They were so scary.' 'They were really critical of me, saying what a pathetic cry-baby I was.' 'They seemed out of control like they would suddenly hit me or shake me.' These give us our fears about others (external fears column); for example, 'people will get angry or shaming if I get upset', 'People are very critical', 'People are more powerful than me', 'People can be scary and unpredictable'.

So, if you had learned to become scared of expressing particular emotions, what did you do, consciously or unconsciously, to make sure that you kept your emotions from coming out? These will go in the 'safety strategies' column. They might include: use my self-critic to have a go at me if I got angry or wanted to cry, stuff the feelings down with food, scratch my arms, clean.

And then the final column is for the downsides or unintended consequences of these safety strategies.

We will then look at how you work with your formulation once you have completed it.

Reflections and notes: What would you like to take hold of and remember from this section on formulation? What would you like to take forward and try? What might be your next steps?

____

____

____

____

Module 36: Protective factors formulation

The formulation is deliberately focused on the things in our lives that create threat emotions, as these are what cause us the most difficulties. However, it is also important to spend some time 'switching systems' into what buffers and has buffered us through our lives. This can take the form of something like a 'protective factors' formulation. This type of formulation would include good memories of helpful experiences with others and with ourselves that we can, and do, draw on through our lives. As we now know, we struggle to access these when our threat mind is running the show. So, it can help to do a compassion practice before we do this, or at least a soothing breathing rhythm practice. However, it can often help just to be prompted to think about these positive aspects – this can be enough to act as a bridge into our soothing/safeness system and all the thoughts, memories, images and so on that it gives us access to.

Our protective factors formulation may prompt us to remember small events or brief moments with people that seem to have a disproportionately helpful effect. But our safeness system is so powerful that it doesn't take as much as we might imagine for it to settle. So don't feel you have to look for something huge. It may be something tiny.

> More and more research is demonstrating that we do not need a whole host of people in our lives for us to feel safe and connected. In fact, just one can be enough – so one good neighbour, one good friend, one good teacher, one good midwife or health visitor, etc., can be enough to buffer us even when times are hard. This is how powerful social support is.

It also means that we can be of immense support to others, just by a smile, an action, and so on. Something tiny that we give, perhaps even without thinking too much of it, can have much more positive and long-lasting impact than we might imagine.

Example of a protective factors formulation

People and events in my background that have helped me	Helpful beliefs I have developed about others	Helpful beliefs I have developed about myself	Resources, support and strategies I draw on (from others – external)/ (within myself – internal)	How these help me
Grandmother – accepting and supportive.	There are people that love me and try to help me.	I am loveable and able to be helped by others.	**External** Look outwards to others as well as in to myself. **Internal** Take courage to ask others for help. Look at how I might be able to be a bit like my grandma to others if I can.	Feel I have people around me – makes me feel calm and safe. I have a sense that I can be brave – makes me feel settled in myself. It makes me happy that I try to give others something that helps them if I can.
Teacher – saw my potential and encouraged me.	There are different people in life who try to help me.	There might be all sorts of good things within me that I hadn't realised were there.	**External** I will open myself to others if I can and trust that they will support me if they can. **Internal** I will keep looking for new good things within me throughout my life.	I feel excited to see what comes of life and the people I meet on the way. I feel warm, curious and excited about myself.
Worked hard and got on the training that gave me this job.	There are all these other people who have worked hard and got jobs like these too and I am part of this group.	I am someone who has strength and commitment to stick at something even when it is challenging.	**External** If things get tricky, there are others going through a similar journey who might be able to support and help me. **Internal** Even when things get difficult, I can find a surprising amount of strength and commitment from within myself.	I feel calm and safe and connected to others. I feel steady, strong, and calm when I remember that I have this strength and commitment even when things are challenging.

My protective factors formulation

People and events in my background that have helped me	Helpful beliefs I have developed about others	Helpful beliefs I have developed about myself	Resources, support and strategies I draw on (from others – external)/ (within myself – internal)	How these help me

Reflections and notes on protective factors formulation. What would you like to hold onto and remember from this? What might you want to take forward and try out?

____

____

____

____

Module 37: Now where? Getting out of our loops and developing a new story for ourselves

Once you have filled out your formulation, you will probably read it through and look it over. However, as we saw in 'multiple selves', the mind that we read it through with and view it from will have a significant impact. We are able to look at our formulation through any of our many possible 'selves' or 'parts'.

What might be the impact of reading through your formulation if:

You looked at it through the eyes of your angry self?

Your anxious self?

Your sad self?

____

____

____

Your critical self?

____

____

____

____

As we can see, it is not just the process of doing our formulation that is key – it is how we regard our formulation, and ourselves as the person who is living this formulation.

Our angry self may respond to it with, 'What was the point of taking me through this process? All it does is blame my parents and that doesn't get me anywhere. I am really angry you suggested I do this.'

Our anxious self may say something like, 'Look! I just get stuck in these loops and go round and round. I will never get out of this!'

Our sad self might say, 'If only I had had a better upbringing. I have lost so much in my life.'

Our critical self might respond with, 'Well what a complete mess you've made of your life, haven't you!?'

How might our compassionate self view our formulation? As ever, we need to make sure we have switched into the compassionate self pattern:

- First get into your 'dignified' posture/'body like a mountain' – with feet flat on the floor, hip width apart, shoulders up, back and down. Eyes closed or focused softly on an object.
- Slow down your in breath, bringing it deep into the base of your lungs, and really slow down your out breath. Feel your body becoming more settled and more stable as your breath slows down.

- Bring a warm, kind face, and warm, kind voice to this practice.
- Now allow that compassionate part of you to come to the foreground. Finding that part of you that tries to be as helpful as it can. The part of you that has great strength, commitment and courage. The part of you that has developed real wisdom about the trickiness and struggle of being human, with our brain, genes, emotions, experiences that we didn't choose, a brain built for us through evolution, not by us. Wisdom gathered throughout our lives through our experiences and the people we have encountered on the way.
- Now, first of all, bring your compassionate mind to what you have written in the 'background' column.

How does your compassionate mind feel towards you as it reads about some of what you have experienced in your life?

____

____

____

____

What does your compassionate mind come to understand about you as it reads about the experiences you have had?

____

____

____

____

What words might the compassionate self want to say to you as it reads about what you have been through?

______

______

______

______

- **Now bring your compassionate mind to the 'fears' column.**

How does your compassionate mind feel as it reads about the fears you experienced?

______

______

______

______

What does your compassionate mind think as it reads about your external and internal fears?

______

______

______

______

What might your compassionate self want to say to you when it reads about these fears?

______

______

- **Now bring your compassionate mind to the 'safety strategies' column**

How does your compassionate self feel as it reads all the ways you have tried, consciously and unconsciously, throughout your life, to keep yourself safe from what you fear?

What words might your compassionate self want to say to you as it reads about your safety strategies?

- **Now bring your compassionate mind to your 'unintended consequences' column.**

How does your compassionate mind feel as it reads about what has unintentionally happened as you tried to keep yourself safe from these fears over the years?

____

____

What might your compassionate self want to say to you as it reads about these unintended consequences?

____

____

____

____

How does your compassionate self feel towards you, that you have been through all of this, trying to manage this all as best you can?

____

____

____

____

How does it feel for you, to have your compassionate self being with you in this way?

____

____

____

____

This is the first part of compassion – turning towards suffering.

The second part is helping to alleviate and prevent it. So now your compassionate self looks at how it can help you with all of this. Rather than getting caught in the loops of the unintended consequences and how we feel about ourselves (self-to-self relating), which then sets off the fears and so on, instead the compassionate mind helps us to begin to move out of these patterns so we can start to live our lives a little differently.

How might your compassionate mind help you with regard to your:

- **Background** (e.g. finding out more about it from others, getting different perspectives, finding out about the wider influences, e.g. the culture it happened in, the background of the people involved)

- **Fears:**

  External (e.g. Looking wider to see if these things are true for all those in your life. Who are the exceptions? If there are people who are also made up of parts that you do value, as well as parts that you struggle with.)

Internal (e.g. Noticing how you would be with your child or someone dear to you if they experienced these fears. How you might wish that key people in your life had been when you had these fears. How it might feel if they had been this way with you. How you might bring these to yourself more and more. How you might ask others, with greater clarity, just what they could do to help you when you experience these fears.)

- **Safety strategies** (e.g. instead of these strategies, what strategies might help you to become more the person you would like to be and get closer to the life you would like to live? How might your compassionate mind help you with the fact that we are wired to have 'better safe than sorry strategies', so taking the steps to try something knew may well be scary? e.g. tiny steps, just holding it in your mind and thinking about it for a while before taking any steps, supporting you if it doesn't go as well as you hoped, encouraging you to try again when you are ready. How might it help you with safety strategies that feel hard to let go of?)

- **Unintended consequences** (e.g. helping you to relate to yourself with compassion that these happen. How to help you to start addressing these in a different way. Helping you with interpreting these in a different way using wisdom, strength, kindness, caring and compassion. Helping you to take the courage to talk to others about what happens and seeing if they can offer thoughts and help.)

What ideas might have arisen from using your compassionate mind with your formulation about ways forward from here? These may be some areas that you would like to make changes to:

Relationship with partner

Relationship with baby

Relationship with parents/friends/at work

My overall plan for how I want to begin to live my life

Ideas for the next few weeks

Ideas for the next few months

Ideas for the next few years

You might find it helpful to collect ideas, thoughts and strategies over the years and put them in your compassionate mind folder or box, e.g. pictures, techniques, phrases, poems, courses, YouTube videos, lists of people who might help, activities you want to try: Something like 'my resource pack / feeding my compassionate mind throughout my life'. There is also space for some in the back of this book.

Reflections and notes: What would you like to take hold of and remember from this section on how we move forward using our formulation? What would you like to take forward and try? What might be your next steps?

Module 38: My partner's formulation

You might want to try to work out what your partner might include for their own formulation, or perhaps go through this together. It can be illuminating and helpful to see how both formulations interact with each other, and what might help you both move forward together, given what you both now know and understand about each other.

How our formulations connect, e.g. what drew us both together, or safety strategies that inadvertently set off the fears of the other person

Aspects of my partner's formulation that I want to particularly remember

How my partner and I can help each other now we know this

How we can use this knowledge to help us be with and bring up our baby

Any other notes

Reflections on working with your partner's formulation; what you would like to hold onto and remember. Anything you would like to both take forward.

Reflections and notes: What would you like to take hold of and remember from this section on your partner's formulation and how both your formulations interconnect? What would you like to take forward and try? What might be your next steps?

My partner's formulation:

Background	Fears		Safety strategies	Unintended consequences
(Key events in your life, particularly relationships)	(What fears or worries your experiences gave you about others (external fears) or yourself (internal fears)		(Conscious or unconscious ways of making sure these fears didn't happen again)	(The downsides of these safety strategies)
	External fears (Others are . . .)	**Internal fears** (I am . . .)		

				Self-to-self relating (How I feel about myself when these unintended consequences happen – these often leave me feeling the very thing I fear, which then sets off my safety strategies and then the unintended consequences get caught in a loop)

Module 39: Working with our inner critic

So far throughout this book, our inner critic (self-critic) has been mentioned many times. For many of us our inner critic is never far away and will pop up for the slightest reason. We have seen how it can figure as a safety strategy in the formulation section, where it can be very effective at preventing us from behaving in a way that we fear might have difficult consequences. For example, it can keep us feeling beaten down and submissive so that we do not become angry, when being angry had meant we got shamed or shouted at by a parent. It can appear to be helpful to us.

Our inner critic has often been around for a very long time in our lives. In fact, many people say that they have had their inner critic with them for as long as they can remember. And it can become part of our very self-identity so we can be worried about who we would become without it. For some, it can feel like the only reliable and ever-present relationship they have had in their lives. As we are so wired for relationships, it can feel better to have the sense of a presence with us, even if it is critical, rather than feeling we are completely alone.

It might seem obvious that we would like to get rid of our inner critic, but given all of this, we can see that it is often not as straightforward as we might initially imagine. Here is a set of steps that can help us to think about our critic in an illuminating way. It then offers a guide to developing an alternative to our inner critic.

(If it works better for you, see https://overcoming.co.uk/715/resources-to-download for downloadable 'inner critic' forms or use your notebook for the following section.)

Understanding our inner critic

Step One:

Imagine that an envelope comes through the post addressed to you. Inside is a big red button. It says that if you press it, your inner critic will be erased from you forever.

Would you press it?

If yes – why would you press it?

____

____

____

How would you imagine you would feel once you had pressed it?

____

____

____

If no – why would you not press it?

____

____

____

Any other action you might take? e.g. save it for another time

____

____

____

Why might you do this?

____

____

____

When we do this exercise with people, the most common response is that at first people say that they would definitely press the red button and that they would feel free, relieved and happy. But then it doesn't usually take too long before people start to have doubts. Here are some of the fears that people say:

'My critic drives me. If I didn't have it, I would become lazy and never achieve anything.'

'I might not be bothered to look after my baby.'

'My critic stops me from saying horrible things to people.'

'I might get big-headed and become a show-off.'

'I might think that I am better than everyone else.'

'I might let out my anger and start destroying things and people.'

'I won't care about any mistakes I make.'

What fear or fears might you have if you pressed the button and got rid of your inner critic forever?

____

____

____

For each fear, we can follow it through to its conclusion; so, for example, if we take the fear, *'I might say horrible things to people'*, we can then ask ourselves **'And if you said horrible things to people?'**

'Then people wouldn't want to be around me. They would avoid me.'

'And if people avoided you?'

'I would be very lonely.'

'And if you were alone?'

'That is a scary and horrible place to be.'

When we track most of our fears to the end in this manner, it often ends up with aloneness. And we know that being alone is a really primal fear, because for most of our evolutionary life, to be cast out, to be alone, was a great survival risk, and even more so if we were pregnant or had a new baby.

So now we can see that our inner critic has a very significant function for us – we believe that it is protecting us from being cast out, from being alone, from being harmed, or from being harmful for example.

This part of really understanding what we might fear if our inner critic were to disappear is an important part of seeing just why we might resist, at some level, getting rid of our inner critic. If we don't realise its deep significance for us, then any work we might do with the inner critic might be subconsciously derailed because deep down life would feel scarier without it. Instead, we can begin to develop an alternative to our critic which we can run alongside it, putting them both to the test until we feel confident which one can be most helpful to us. Once we know, we can then put our efforts into growing the one that we want to keep.

Step Two:

In Step One, we identified a sense of the function that the inner critic has in our lives. It can give a feeling that it is helping us in some way. In Step Two we will look at this 'helpfulness' in more detail.

Close your eyes and imagine that you have just made a bit of a mistake, nothing too serious. Perhaps you opened the fridge and caught your sleeve on the milk in a hurry and knocked it on the floor, spilling milk all over the place. Or some other mild example from your life that brings the voice of your critic into your head. You might hear something like 'Why are you always so clumsy? You never look properly at what you are doing.'

Imagine that your inner critic could appear in front of you.

What does it look like? (Its size and shape. It might be like a cartoon character or a person or something else entirely. What colour is it?)

____

____

How is it relating to you? (Is it saying anything? How is it being with you?)

____

____

What are the feelings it is directing towards you? How does it seem to feel about you?

____

____

How are you feeling inside when it relates to you in this way? What is the feeling in your body?

____

____

If this feeling were to grow and grow, what would your body really want to do if it could?

____

____

Imagine that it found out about something that you had messed up, or not done well. How would it be with you?

____

____

Imagine that it found out that you had done well at something. How would it be with you?

____

____

Come back into that steady, strong, wise part of you. Feel your body sitting taller and broader; 'like a mountain'. Slow down your breathing. Soften your face and hear your gentle, kind voice in your mind. Take in the sounds around you. Feel your feet on the floor. Feel your seat supporting you. When you are ready, gently open your eyes.

These are some of the things that people have taken from this part of the exercise:

1. Although they may have picked something mild, the critic still felt horrible to be with. Sometimes people are shocked by how scary the critic can be.
2. Some people describe cartoon-type characters, or a type of critical person from a children's film. Others

describe a version of themselves, but one which is tall and thin, being very disappointed in them. There is a whole array of critics.

3. Some are very tall or big in relation to them, others are smaller than them, some the same size.
4. The colours of the critic are often similar; grey, brown, black, dark green, dark red.
5. The feelings the critic has towards people are typically anger, disappointment, contempt, frustration, being so cross that they don't even want to look at them, or they just walk off.
6. The critic might be pointing an angry finger at them, shaking their head slowly in disappointment, shouting at them, raising an eyebrow and saying nothing but suggesting, 'Well, what did you expect? You are useless', or wanting to grab and shake them in frustration.
7. The feelings people often have in their body in the presence of their critic are anxiety, feeling sick, shaky, weak, heart racing. Occasionally people feel angry but usually wouldn't feel able to display that anger or argue back.
8. If the feeling were to grow in the body, people described feeling like they wanted to disappear – 'the ground to swallow me up' – to run away, feeling too shaky to move, feeling frozen to the spot, unable to look at the critic with head down, or looking at the critic in fear.
9. The critic is usually not surprised when they find out that you messed something up. They might act with derision, contempt, a 'Well there you go, what did you expect?' kind of shrug, or more anger, and more frustration.
10. When the critic hears that you did well at something, the critic is still not happy, in fact it can become even more contemptuous; 'What? Do you want a gold medal for that? Well next time you will just mess up like you usually do. This was just luck this time.'

This exercise is often a powerful one. It can demonstrate that we might strive and strive in the hope that our critic will be proud of us or leave us alone. But actually, even when we do well, the critic remains dismissive, contemptuous and critical. This is the nature of the critic. It is generated by the threat system, so its only strategies are those that exist within the threat system – to attack, to scare, to threaten, to put down, using the submissive-dominant or competitive rank system ('one up, one down' system).

At the beginning of this exercise, we looked at what we thought the function of our inner critic was for us. We imagined whether we would press the red button that would extinguish our critic forever, and what our fear might be if we did.

We might have believed that our critic makes us get things done and stops us from being lazy or helps us to do well at work or in parenting our children.

Step Three:

Have a look back at what you believed your critic did for you (at the beginning of this exercise).

Now think about how you felt when your critic appeared in front of you. What was the urge in your body?

____

____

So, did your critic help you to move towards the person you want to be? Did you feel it helped you have the energy and motivation to get on and achieve things? To try again when things get hard? To find ways to improve at work? To become the parent you would like to be?

____

____

What was the impact of the critic on you?

____

____

We might be starting to see that our critic doesn't work quite as we thought. And in fact, because our critic is never happy, no matter how well we do, we can begin to feel hopeless and helpless. As it is inside of us, we can never escape it either, even in the night. Indeed, our critic can cause us to feel anxious and depressed and sometimes even suicidal.

Step Four:

Imagine that you have a friend or a loved one, or your child when they are older, who is struggling with something. Perhaps they are struggling with reading. You are trying to find somebody who could give them some extra help.

Would you pick your critic?

If so, why?

If not, why not?

Whom would you pick instead? What qualities would you be looking for in them?

Usually, people realise that although they have this critic for themselves, they would never pick anybody like this to help someone they cared about. Or if they would, usually they would have some conditions – 'Perhaps not as harsh as my one, but I wouldn't want them to be given too easy a time of it. I want them to actually get better at reading', for example.

So, what qualities do people say that they would want this person to have who was helping someone they cared about to become better at reading?

Here are some of the qualities that people list:

- Encouraging
- Looking at mistakes and identifying what they are doing wrong and how to help them get it right
- Enthusiastic
- Listening
- Identifying what would help this particular person
- Empathy
- Humour
- Kindness
- Warmth
- Having the strength to keep on going even when things get trickier
- Really wanting the best for that person
- Wisdom – understanding their subject well, what helps and hinders people to learn, the nature of being human, own life experiences

What people end up describing is a list of qualities that make up a compassionate person or being.

What other qualities would you want this person to have?

____

____

____

____

What difference might it have made in your life if such a person had been there for you?

____

____

How might they help you when things get difficult with your baby?

Which qualities would you like to have available in your baby's life? (List as many as you wish.)

Not all qualities exist in any one person. If you could bring together a team of people for your baby, who would be in that team? (It can be anyone – their grandma, a health visitor, a next-door neighbour, you, your partner . . . They don't have to be alive or even real. They could be characters from books or films or children's cartoons, for example.)

Reflections: What are the things that particularly struck you about this exercise?

What aspects would you like to make a note of to remember from this exercise?

____

____

____

____

Compassionate teacher (parent/guide/coach) versus 'nice' teacher

Many people can remember, or know, a teacher who wanted to be a 'nice' teacher. Often children have very little respect for such teachers, which can seem puzzling and of course awful for that teacher. This lack of respect can arise because the children realise, at some level, that the teacher is coming from a place of threat and submission. Rather than focusing on the children, they are focused on themselves and how to ensure that they are liked and not attacked. This is not the teacher's fault, and if they were to do their own formulation, in all likelihood we would see why this safety strategy of 'being nice' is completely understandable.

Now think of a teacher who was an inspiration. Perhaps they made a significant and positive difference to your life or to someone else's. They might also initially be described as 'nice' too, but with a subtle difference. That subtle difference is in the focus of their attention. Sometimes they may even come across as quite strict or a bit scary initially. But what children pick up is that the teacher's focus is on trying to really help the children to flourish and become the best of themselves. The teacher doesn't particularly care if they are liked or not – it is not about them, it is about the children. They are the kind of teachers who might make you do your work again when they know you really didn't do your best, or go the extra mile for you, perhaps spending some of their lunch time with you to help you get to grips with something.

This is where we see the importance of the strength, courage and wisdom of the compassionate mind. These teachers are not 'soft' or just 'nice'. They will tell you when you have made a mistake or upset somebody or are becoming 'lazy' – but in a way that is understanding and helpful. They are somebody you can trust, because their intention is to be as helpful to you as they can, even if it means they must bear your initial annoyance at them. They are doing this in the best interests of you, not themselves.

Our compassionate self or compassionate being acts as our guide, teacher, mentor and coach.
We can trust in it to be helpful, rather than just say what we want to hear so that we like it.
It has the courage and strength to be able to say and do the things it does
even if this is sometimes very hard.
Its presence helps us to feel safe in the world;
knowing that even when things are the most difficult they can be,
they are standing by us, with strength, courage, wisdom
and a deep intention to help us no matter what.

Reflections and notes: What would you like to take hold of and remember from this section on working with your inner critic and developing a compassionate teacher, guide or coach as an alternative? What would you like to take forward and try? What might be your next steps?

___

___

___

___

Module 40: Compassionate versus critical thinking

As we covered earlier in the book, rather than aiming to remove or destroy the inner critic, the compassionate mind approach aims to build an alternative inner pattern; one of compassion. We also discussed how our inner critic has often been with us for most of our lives so the thought of it suddenly disappearing can be worrying. Instead, the focus of the work shifts to building the inner compassionate self and then beginning to test it out in the world. Ultimately, we would bring our compassionate mind to understanding our inner critic and perhaps working with it to help it settle. Just like learning to swim, we don't usually do this by leaping into the deep end. Instead, we might hang on to the side of the shallow end with our feet able to touch the bottom and start to practise a few tentative swimming strokes. We do that with the compassionate self too. It means we can practise it, try it out and tweak it and change it as we need to.

We are only likely to persist with the compassionate mind approach if we start to see its benefits. This exercise can be a helpful one to begin practising our compassionate self, as well as seeing whether it is indeed making a difference to us.

(This form can be downloaded from https://overcoming.co.uk/715/resources-to-download)

Event	Inner critic's response	How this made me feel (0 = 'terrible,' 10 = 'really good')	Compassionate mind's response (Switch systems – 'Body like a mountain, breath like the wind, mind like the sky,' warm, kind face and voice)	How this made me feel (0 = 'terrible', 10 = 'really good')
My baby wouldn't stop crying in the café	'*Everybody is looking at you thinking what a useless parent you are. They are getting really annoyed with you for ruining their lunch and they are wondering why you are not hurrying up and getting out.*'	Rating-1 I felt so ashamed and embarrassed. I don't think I could go in that café ever again. I am not sure I want to go out with my baby anymore if that is going to happen.	*'Oh, it is horrible when this happens. You tried so hard to make sure your baby would be OK before you came out. But this is just what babies do. It isn't their fault, and it isn't your fault. What makes it harder is that our brains are wired to need people to think well of us, even more so when we have a baby. And that is on top of your background of learning to please people to keep them close. None of this is your fault. It just makes this extra hard. All of the people here have been children themselves and most will have had children and know what you are going through. Just do your best and perhaps connect with those around you, e.g. saying with ease and warmth, "Sorry about all this noise. I thought we'd manage a nice peaceful lunch but she's just not having it today."'*	Rating-5 I still feel a bit rattled by this, but I am designed to be rattled when my baby cries and when I think I have bothered other people. Particularly in the perinatal time when we need others even more. I will just go home and get my baby and myself sorted out and we can have a cup of tea at home and do something nice together. Anyhow, I am sure this will be something to share with people when I see them next.

Your example

Event	Inner critic's response	How this made me feel (0 = 'terrible,' 10 = 'really good')	Compassionate mind's response (Switch systems – 'Body like a mountain, breath like the wind, mind like the sky,' warm, kind face and voice)	How this made me feel (0 = 'terrible', 10 = 'really good')

Imagine that a really kind, wise, strong, caring being has turned up. They might be your compassionate other/being or they might be a new image. Now imagine that they read out column four to you (the compassionate mind's response) slowly in their kind, warm voice.

How do you feel? What rating would you put in column five now?

____

____

____

Anything else that you noticed?

____

____

____

____

When we do the compassionate thinking exercise, we can often do it more in our head, using logic and knowledge. It can be helpful. However, when we imagine a warm, kind, compassionate being with us, we have now switched on a whole set of social safeness systems within us, including the vagus nerve, which make us feel safe, calm and understood. This enables us to really take in and feel the message that the compassionate being is giving us.

It is as if hearing and seeing this warm, kind being enables us to soak in the compassionate message rather than having it just slide off us.

When you imagine your compassionate self or your compassionate image talking to you, deliberately slow down your voice,

and bring warmth and kindness to your face and to your voice tone.

This enables the compassion to soak in rather than slide off us.

Reflections and notes: What would you like to take hold of and remember from this section on compassionate versus critical thinking? What would you like to take forward and try? What might be your next steps?

___

___

___

___

Module 41: The compassionate letter

Many of the techniques used in compassionate mind training involve imagery. Compassionate writing is a very different way of switching on and strengthening the compassion system. It can be helpful for those who find imagery difficult, but even those who find imagery relatively easy can find that compassionate letter writing brings a different and very powerful dimension to the compassionate mind.

Often people who find writing difficult, who don't enjoy it, or associate it in a negative way with school and being 'marked', for example, are understandably wary of compassionate letter writing, but if they persevere, it often surprises people by its helpfulness. It is worth giving it a go and seeing what comes of it for you.

There is no pressure to get it right, spell it properly, have it make sense, make it good, or write a lot; this is just for you.

- Take a piece of paper and a pen or pencil.
- Sit somewhere you feel comfortable.
- We are going to firstly go through a short compassionate mind practice to help you shift systems, and to make sure you are in your compassionate mind as best you can. Then at the end you will just open your eyes, let your compassionate mind pick up your pen or pencil and begin writing to you.
- Close your eyes or allow your eyes to relax and gently focus on an object.
- Sit back in your seat, upright and with your feet resting on the floor, hip width apart.
- Bring your shoulders up to your ears and drop them back and down. Feel the openness in your body.
- Bring your warm, kind face, and warm, kind voice to this practice, perhaps imagine welcoming yourself here, saying 'Hello!' and your name.
- Now bring your warm, kind face and voice to your breath, perhaps imagining greeting it warmly now you are spending a short while with it ('Hello breath!').
- Begin slowing down your in breath, bringing it smoothly and deeply into the base of

your lungs, feeling the pause, then really slowing down your out breath, perhaps in your mind saying, 'breath, slowing, down'.

- As your breath begins to slow, you might notice your body begin to settle, and feel more steady, more stable.
- Now bring to mind your compassionate image or being, or an idea of a compassionate being, or the part of you that really wants to be as helpful as it can. The being or part that has a wise understanding that humans have a particular brain and body, set up and shaped for them by nature and by their experiences, which can do amazing things but also make being human very difficult for us, and that this isn't our fault. This part also has great strength of character, and courage, and can do difficult things.
- Feeling the warmth, kindness and understanding of this compassionate being, or your compassionate self, they would like to write you a letter. It may be about something specific or just writing to you about how things are for you in general.
- Now open your eyes. This wise, strong, kind, understanding being or part is now going to pick up the pen or pencil and begin writing to you. They might start 'Dear . . . ' and your name. Write for as long as you wish but see if you can write for at least ten minutes. Write from your 'heart' rather than your 'head'.

Dear ____________________________

____

____

____

____

____

____

____

____

____

- When you feel your compassionate mind has finished writing to you, read your letter through. Change or add anything, particularly in any areas where the critic has crept in. Our body is usually very good at picking up how our letter feels to us.

How do you feel as you read your letter through?

- Once you have made any changes, read it again (it can be very powerful to read it aloud, or to have someone read it to you). This time really focus on reading it very slowly with a warm, kind voice tone and facial expression.

How do you feel? Does it feel different to when you read it through the first time?

What things particularly struck you about this?

Did you cover any of these areas? If not, add them in and see how the letter feels now:

- **Engagement with suffering**:

  1. Care for wellbeing (your motivation, intention and heartfelt wish for yourself): e.g. *'I wanted to write to you because I can see that you have been having such a difficult time since Baby was born. I wanted to let you know that I am here with you and to help you as best I can.'*

Your examples of communicating your wish or hope for yourself with this letter

____

____

____

____

  2. Sensitivity to the distress (seeing all the areas of suffering): e.g. *'I can see that you have been waking feeling so anxious and full of dread, and you have been trying to hide this from everyone which is putting such a strain on you. This has been so very hard for you.'*

Your examples of demonstrating your sensitivity to your distress

____

____

____

____

  3. Sympathy (being moved by the suffering): e.g. *'I am so sorry that you have been going through all of this. I know that you were so looking forward to having a baby, and you are so disappointed with how things have turned out so far. I can feel just how painful this is for you.'*

Your examples of sympathy for yourself

4. Distress tolerance (being able to bear the feelings that come up): e.g. *'Although your feelings of disappointment and sadness are painful, they will pass, as all feelings do, and in the meantime you can use all your usual strategies that have helped you get through painful feelings in the past, and the new ones you have been discovering too; your compassion practice, going and doing things that you enjoy with your baby even though you are feeling this way, spending time with people you feel comfortable with . . .'*

Your examples of distress tolerance you might want to put in this letter to yourself

5. Empathy (understanding just why this is significant to you as opposed to anyone else): e.g. *'This is so particularly hard for you because you really wanted this baby, and you also have learned to set very high standards for yourself in order to feel loved and accepted. You wanted people to be proud of you when you became a mum, but now you feel you have let them down. This is so painful, and scary, because you really do want, and need, their help too.'*

Your examples of how you might be empathic to yourself in this letter

6. Non-judgement (understanding and accepting that these feelings and issues are part of human suffering. Holding them with warmth and kindness without being critical or judgemental of them):
   e.g. '*These struggles and feelings are common, and normal, if very painful, aspects of having a new baby, and have been experienced the world over for hundreds of years. These are not your fault at all.*'

Your examples of conveying non-judgement to yourself in your letter

Some ideas around compassionate letter writing that people have found helpful:

- Try this at different times and for different issues. People often find that the experience can deepen if you have a few goes at this.
- Try writing it from your compassionate self and then your compassionate being or image and see if there is a difference.
- Put it in an envelope and post it to yourself. It can be extraordinarily powerful to receive it in the post.
- Write on a postcard to yourself – the small size of it can feel easier.
- Write to your baby.
- Write to you and your baby (Dear [your name] and [Baby's name]). Particularly if you have been through a difficult birth together or you and your baby had a difficult start together.
- Write a fairy story to your baby.
- Write to your partner.

- Write a poem.
- Put your letter in a place where you will find it in the future, e.g. in your summer shorts or winter jumper.
- There are websites where you can write a compassionate letter and have it posted to you in the future.
- You can stick your letter in the back of the book in your resources section so you can find it when you need it.
- Or add any words or sentences that pop into your mind over the weeks, months, even years, that you would like to say to yourself, to the resources section at the back of the book. These will be there for whenever you need them in the future.
- Also add words and sentences that you might want to remember that you have said to others, others have said to you, or that you come across in any circumstance, e.g. in books, online, or overheard in the supermarket queue.

Reflections and notes: What would you like to take hold of and remember from this section on compassionate letter writing? What would you like to take forward and try? What might be your next steps?

____

____

____

____

Module 42: Compassionate attention versus critical attention

Another very powerful way of strengthening our compassionate mind, whilst also bringing further clarity to just how it differs from our critical mind, is by understanding the nature of attention. Ironically, attention is something we might not pay much attention to. Our attention is usually guided for us by our mind, and as we now know, our threat mind will have the strongest hold over it. But once we know how our attention can affect us, we might then want to take more conscious charge of where it goes.

The nature of attention

Exercise One:

- Bring to mind a really nice trip to the park or trip out that you have had – it might be a recent one, or one further back in time. It might not be clear in your mind; just a sense and a feel of it is enough.

What was it that made it so nice?

____

____

How do you feel as you remember it?

____

____

What is happening in your body?

____

What thoughts are coming to mind?

- Now bring to mind a trip to the park or trip out that wasn't so great. Nothing too severe; perhaps it wasn't particularly nice weather, or it was a bit too busy for example.

What was it that meant it wasn't so great?

How do you feel as you remember it?

What is happening in your body?

What thoughts are coming to mind?

____

____

- Now go back to the really nice trip and bring that to mind again. Allow it to really soak into your body as if it was warmth from the sun, or a hot water bottle.

How does that make you feel?

____

____

Although we were moving our attention back and forth between memories quite quickly, you may have found that they had very different effects on your images, thoughts, feelings, and body. All we did was direct the spotlight of our attention from one type of memory to another, yet it affected the whole of us. And it can carry on affecting us after the memory has gone, as it has switched the pattern we are in (here we moved from the pattern we were in already, to joy or pleasure, then to threat, and then back to joy again) and the pattern we are in will affect the next thing we do.

This is helpful to know if we would like to be able to choose the pattern we are in, rather than letting our mind just do it for us (although mostly it still will – this is just the nature of our human set-up, but we can train our brain to become better and better at switching our attention).

This next exercise can help to deepen our understanding of the nature of attention even further.

Exercise Two:

- Close your eyes. Direct your attention as if it is like a spotlight or torchlight, onto your left big toe.

What do you notice? (You might notice the feel of your toe against your sock or footwear or resting on the floor. You might notice sensations inside your toe. Or perhaps you don't notice anything at all – that is still noticing something.)

- Now move the spotlight of attention to shine on your right big toe.

What do you notice?

- Now move your attention to the feel of your left hand resting on your leg.

What do you notice? (Perhaps the weight of your hand on your leg, the feel of the contact between your hand and your leg, perhaps sensations inside your hand or your leg, or maybe nothing at all.)

- Now move your attention to your lips.

What do you notice? (You might notice the feel of your lips against your teeth, the feel of the air on your lips, sensations within your lips, or again perhaps nothing at all.)

- Now open your eyes.

What struck you about this exercise? What will you take from it?

____

____

These are some of the things that people have noticed with this little exercise:

- When you focused on one part of the body the other parts seemed to disappear. And that other things you may have been attending to seem to disappear too, such as sounds or thoughts that were previously coming into your mind.
- The things that you focus on seem to expand in size (some people say that their lips feel bigger, for example) and certainly fill up our attention.
- As ever, the threat or critical mind can be close by, creating thoughts such as 'Am I doing this right?', 'What is wrong with my toe?'
- It can be hard moving your attention sometimes – some people noticed wanting to stay with the left big toe for example and resisted moving on to the right big toe.

In terms of the compassionate mind approach, this exercise shows us that wherever we direct our attention will become the focus of our attention; everything else seems to vanish. Applying this to the three circles; if we focus on something that triggers our threat system then that is what is going to fill our mind. The other circles, drive and soothing, and even our compassionate mind which guides our three circles, seem to disappear. But as we know from the exercise, our toes don't disappear just because we aren't focused on them, and it is the same with the soothing system or the compassionate mind; they are still there. We just need to draw our attention to them to stimulate them, then they become the focus of our attention.

And as we saw from attending to different memories – it isn't just that different things fill our attention, they also have an impact on our body, our thoughts, our behaviour, our images and the memories we recall. It is quite incredible really and so helpful to realise.

When we are building our compassionate mind

we need to deliberately focus our attention on aspects that stimulate it.

Even when we think we have lost it, or that we never had it, it is just that it has dropped into the shadows.

We just need to shine a light on it again.

And we can use this nature of our attention to help us to switch systems from threat to soothing if we wish.

However, as we may have seen even in the above exercise, the threat system is very powerful and can hold our attention like a magnet, or pull our attention back to it when we have moved it away. This is how attention is designed to be – it is a survival strategy that has remained in humans because it works. So, we need to be kind and understanding to ourselves when we try to shift our attention from threat to soothing but find we struggle. That is not our fault.

Here are some examples which help us to compare the different impacts of focusing on threat versus compassion focused aspects. (Don't forget, for the compassion focus column you need to switch systems from threat to soothing – use the five stepping stones – 'dignified' posture, slowing down your breath, warm kind face and voice and then talk to yourself slowly as if a kind, wise, strong, caring compassionate person is talking to you.)

(This form can be downloaded from https://overcoming.co.uk/715/resources-to-download)

Aspect we are attending to	Threat focus	My thoughts	How I feel	Compassion focus (Switch systems – 'Body like a mountain, breath like the wind, mind like the sky', warm, kind face and voice)	My thoughts	How I feel
Out walking in rain with my baby in their buggy.	*My wet feet.* *My cold hands.* *How far is it to home?*	*I wish I hadn't come out. What a silly thing to do.*	*Miserable and fed up.*	*My baby has enjoyed the change of scenery, and they are warm and dry.* *I have enjoyed getting out even though it's wet and cold.* *The rain looks beautiful on the leaves.* *I can't wait to bring out my baby in their wellington boots when they are older to jump in the puddles. They will love it.*	*I am glad I did this, for me and for my baby. It has helped me to see that my baby loves being outside whatever the weather and I am pleased about that.*	*Quite joyful really despite the rain.*

Going to playgroup.	*The people not talking to me.* *The people looking when my baby cries.*	*No-one wants to talk to me.* *They are thinking I am a rubbish mother.*	*Lonely, anxious and ashamed.*	*The people that are smiling at me.* *The people looking as scared as me.* *My baby enjoying being here.*	*There are people who want me to feel welcomed and there are people who feel just as anxious and who want to make friends but are scared of being rejected just like me.* *It's not surprising I am finding this hard; coming somewhere on your own is a hard thing to do, especially when you are shy and self-critical. But actually my baby is really enjoying seeing everyone and having different toys to play with. I am pleased I can do that for my baby.*	*Calmer, reassured, a little bit proud of myself actually. I have more strength and courage than I realised.*

Your example:

Aspect we are attending to	Threat focus	My thoughts	How I feel	Compassion focus (Switch systems – 'Body like a mountain, breath like the wind, mind like the sky', warm, kind face and voice)	My thoughts	How I feel

Exercise: This is one that you can fill in focused on your baby

Aspect we are attending to	Threat focus	My thoughts	How I feel	Compassion focus (Switch systems – 'Body like a mountain, breath like the wind, mind like the sky', warm, kind face and voice)	My thoughts	How I feel
My baby's skin	*Dry scaly patches and some nappy rash.*	*I haven't really been caring for my baby well enough.* *People are going to see these and judge me for my poor parenting.*	*Horrible, ashamed, anxious.*	*The lovely smooth parts of my baby's skin.* *The fact that I am keeping an eye on the rash and I am trying different things to make it better. I won't be just ignoring it.* *Seeing that other babies have all this too – it is very normal.*	*I can enjoy my baby just as they are – literally the rough with the smooth.* *I feel reassured when I remind myself that this is all normal and I am doing my best for my baby.*	*Reassured, calm, joy.*

My baby's behaviour.	*They get grumbly during the day.* *Crying when we are out in public.* *Wanting to go to their dad rather than me.*	*I am no good at being a mother. Everyone can see this too and will be looking down on me.*	*Ashamed, alone, sad, anxious, sometimes a bit angry at my baby and my partner.*	*My baby being happy and contented during the day.* *My baby being curious and interested in me and the world around them.* *The times my baby comes to me rather than others.*	*It is very painful when my baby wants to go to dad rather than me and I need to support myself with the suffering I am in rather than criticising and shaming myself. I think I will talk to my partner about it.* *Actually, though, things are going pretty well really. My baby gets tired, bored, uncomfortable, like we all do, and they know to let me know about it so I can help them.* *My baby looks to me for comfort but also enjoys being with other people too and that is really what I want for my baby.*	*Calmer, happy, pleased, proud, joyful.*

Your baby focused examples:

Aspect we are attending to	Threat focus	My thoughts	How I feel	Compassion focus (Switch systems – 'Body like a mountain, breath like the wind, mind like the sky', warm, kind face and voice)	My thoughts	How I feel
Your baby focused examples:						

Exercise: What I have done all day

Aspect we are attending to	Threat focus	My thoughts	How I feel	Compassion focus (Switch systems – 'Body like a mountain, breath like the wind, mind like the sky', warm kind face and voice)	My thoughts	How I feel
My baby	*Times I was slow to respond to my baby.* *Times they cried.*	*I am really no good at this.*	*Down, ashamed, defeated.*	*The times I watch to check they are OK. The times I respond quickly.* *Sitting holding my baby* *Sitting feeding my baby.* *Taking my baby out.* *Talking to my baby.*	*I really am focused on my baby such a lot; much more than I realised. I spend such a lot of my day holding them in mind, looking after them, trying to help them have a good day.*	*Warm inside, happy, calm, pleased, motivated.*
Your examples:						

The house **Your examples:**	*The washing that needs doing.* *The mess that needs clearing up.* *The baby things that are cluttering the house.* *The things that need fixing.*	*It is all a total mess and chaos. I cannot keep on top of all of this.* *No-one can come round otherwise they will see that I am just not coping.*	*Down, a failure, ashamed, anxious, a bit angry, sad for my old life which I felt I was relatively good at.*	*All the evidence that there is now a precious baby in our lives.* *The tininess of the clothes.* *The room we got ready for our baby.* *All the things that we have bought or made for our baby.* *All the things other people have bought or made for our baby.*	*It is quite incredible that there is a whole person living in our house who didn't exist before – what a joy and a wonder.* *We have really put a lot into making a space for this baby that will make them comfortable and happy.* *Other people have welcomed them into this life too.*	*Joy, wonder, warmth, happiness, safe, connected to others.*

My partner						
Other people						
Myself						

The future							
Anything else:							

Your reflections on this section. What would you like to hold onto and remember? Anything you want to take forward and put into action?

____

____

____

____

The maternal brain and attention

We have discussed earlier in the book the degree to which pregnancy changes the brain. The process of caring and interacting regularly with a baby also changes the brain of those closely interacting with the person who is pregnant and the baby once it is born.

Our attention is governed by the motivational system that we are in. If we are hungry then the motivational system concerned with finding food gets switched on. Our brain will hyperfocus on looking for food. It can be hard to focus on anything else. If our motivation is to compete then our focus of attention will be on making sure we are winning or are the best. The brain changes that we see during pregnancy seem to be about really turning up our focus on the baby and our feelings of delight and reward when we attend to them. It switches on our care-giving motivational system. (Our baby will have its care-*receiving* motivational system switched on.) However, 'being maternal' is not just about delighting in and directly nurturing our baby. From an evolutionary point of view, it is also about doing whatever it takes to keep our child alive until they are able to reproduce. So 'maternal behaviour' might be about making alliances, lying, cheating, scheming, competing to get food or protection for our baby. And for most of our evolutionary life as humans, mothers would have been having to make painful choices in terms of which of their children to keep alive if resources were limited.

So, in terms of maternal attention, it may be that we become focused on holding our baby in mind but also holding any threat there too, and working out what it will take to best keep our baby alive. 'Maternal behaviour' through the ages may not fit at all with the 'Madonna' archetype of motherhood. In fact, we can see that it is only recently in human history, and still only in reasonably safe and well-resourced countries, that we can entertain the 'luxury' of aspiring to the Madonna archetype of an endlessly loving, calm mother who gives equal resources to all her children.

Have there been any changes in what draws your attention that have particularly surprised you since having a baby?

____

____

Have you noticed any changes in what draws your partner's attention that have surprised your partner/you/both?

____

____

The brain changes in particular ways and, as we saw before, it seems to change in ways to do with the baby as we might expect, but also in ways concerning our relationships with others around us, as we are also wired to need to share the care of our baby.

This means that the process of pregnancy and parenthood will be having an impact on our attention, regardless of whether we would like it to.

As we are wired to need others to share in the care of our baby, we are also likely to find that our attention to our relationships with others and whether we and our baby are held positively in mind by others, is also turned up. This may account for why, for example, the pregnant brain focuses us more on the emotions in others as pregnancy progresses.

An observed change in a mother's attention when she becomes pregnant has been termed 'maternal preoccupation', describing the turning inwards of her attention to the baby inside her. This becomes intensified when the baby begins to move and particularly when they respond to external and internal stimuli. A mother's shift in attention may be very noticeable to others, particularly where what may have preoccupied her before is no longer such a pull. This may include her job, friends without children, and values she held dear which no longer seem so important. There can also be strong attentional pulls to 'nesting', and in looking more critically at where the baby will live, to the extent that moving house whilst heavily pregnant is not uncommon.

The brain may draw our focus to ourselves and our health as parents and protectors of our baby, and we may find we become more preoccupied with health anxiety. As mentioned before, women also report an increase in attention to wanting their mum, or an ideal of a mum they wished they had. This may be in response to the evolved role of the grandmother in improving the survival chances of her daughter and grandchild if she is involved in sharing the care.

There are many ways in which our brain and our biology will be guiding our attention now we have a baby, as these have been wired into us by nature to maximise the chances of keeping our child alive. These can be perturbing and confusing as the person we thought we were can really change once we have a baby, but this is not our fault. We can, however, learn to hold all of this with our compassionate mind, and use it to support us and guide us through all of these changes. After all, if some major event had happened to our brain, such as a brain injury, then we would receive a great deal of support and be expected to need time to adapt and reorganise and consolidate our new brain, abilities and sense of self. With parenthood we have a major brain change and then have a new baby to look after. So being held with a compassionate mind, by ourselves and others, is crucial at this time.

Practice: Mindfulness to attention

- Close your eyes or settle your gaze gently on an object.
- Sit upright in your 'dignified' posture, feet flat on the floor, hip width apart. Bring your shoulders up to your ears, drop them back and down.
- Allow your jaw and your tongue to relax.
- Bring your warm, kind face and warm, kind voice to your breath. Perhaps greeting it warmly, 'Hello breath!'
- Slow down your in breath, bringing it smoothly and deeply into the base of your lungs, feel the pause, then really slow down your out breath. Perhaps in your mind on your next out breath saying, 'Breath, slowing, down'. And then on the next out breath saying in your mind, 'Body, slowing, down'.

- You might notice a sense of your body becoming steadier and sturdier.
- Move into the 'blue sky' of your mind, so that you are just sitting quietly observing all that flows across it as if they are clouds passing by.
- You might notice your mind listening to sounds, then moving to sensations in your body, then shifting to thoughts, and so on.
- Watch from this calm, steady, curious place whatever floats in and out of your attention.
- You may well get caught up in something. Perhaps your mind gets carried away by one thought after another. When you notice this, come back to your mindful position, as if you are sitting on a bank of a river, watching leaves floating by.
- Another analogy is of sitting watching cars and buses go by. Getting caught up in thoughts or sensations or sounds is like suddenly finding you have got on a bus. As soon as you notice, get off and return to just sitting watching the cars and buses going by.
- When your mind does get caught up ('falls in the river' or 'gets on a bus'), guide your mind gently and kindly back to this place of observing (i.e. the 'blue sky mind', 'on the river bank', 'back next to the road observing the cars and buses'.)
- From this place of open awareness observe whatever flows in and out of it once again.
- You might become aware of the nature of attention; for example, how quickly or slowly it moves from one focus to another, what particularly holds your attention for longer, what feels easier to shift attention from, what happens to aspects that seem to have held your attention strongly for a while.
- Notice what shifts your attention to deciding to end the session. See if you can sit and attend to this and to what your mind does with this. See if you can sit beyond this decision and see what happens to your attention.
- When you are ready, shift your attention to the sense of you back here in the room. Notice the sounds coming in through your ears. Feel the sensation of your chair steady underneath you. Notice the feel of your feet in contact with the floor, perhaps moving them. Notice the feel of your hands, perhaps flexing and moving them.

- Then gently open your eyes. See if you can take this calm awareness into the next part of your day.

End of practice.

Your reflections and notes on this practice. What would you like to take hold of and remember from this section on the nature of attention, the impact of becoming a mother on attention, and compassionate versus critical attention? What would you like to take forward and try? What might be your next steps?

____

____

____

____

____

Module 43: Compassionate behaviour

As with our attention, our thinking, our imagery and our memories when we are in a pattern of threat, how we behave towards ourselves and others and what we set off to do can be very different compared to when we are in a pattern of compassion.

With a new baby in our life, what we are doing may look a world away from what we were doing before our baby came along. We are having to learn, adapt, pay attention in particular ways, keep going day, and night, caring for our baby, and ourselves, and anyone else in our family, as best we can. When it is challenging, when we are exhausted, when we doubt ourselves, when we feel frustrated, then the many actions and behaviours we engage in come from a pattern of threat – anger, anxiety, the self-critic. This is not our fault, just the way our brain and body work.

Often, we behave in these ways without even realising why, or that we might be able to do something different. Sometimes the influences on our behaviour stem not from all that comes of having a new baby, but from our life before our baby – perhaps our relationship with our partner, or factors to do with where we live, or the culture we are parenting in. It may be that the influences on our behaviour go way back and have accompanied us through our lives or have been brought into existence by having a baby. Putting these behaviours into our formulation can be really enlightening in helping us to understand just why we might find ourselves behaving in this way. Whatever the cause, rarely do we wake up with the intention that today's aim is to make this a really horrible day for ourselves and others. So as with all aspects of ourselves, we need to change the pattern of our mind and body from one of threat to one of compassion – then the behaviour that flows from this will be behaviour that is supported by an intention of trying to be as helpful as we can, to ourselves, and to others.

Compassionate behaviour is about what will help us with any suffering that we have now, or may have in the future, and also what helps us to grow and flourish. It also takes joy in us too. We might need compassionate behaviour to help us in this current moment, or to help us in the next weeks, months or years.

Examples of compassionate behaviour in the moment

- Putting your baby safely in their cot while you go out of the room to take a breather and calm down.
- Choosing to make a cup of tea and watch the birds whilst baby sleeps to help recharge a bit rather than doing some jobs.
- Making gentle, warm eye contact with other people at the baby group.
- Standing up tall, in your 'dignified' pose, slowing your breath, and softening your face and voice to help swap patterns, even though you feel angry or anxious.
- Picking your baby up and soothing them when they are upset.
- Helping your baby with something new when they get bored.
- Feeding your baby when they get hungry.
- Keeping an eye on your baby to make sure they are safe and OK.
- Despite being tired yourself, wanting to remember to ask your partner about something they've been worried about.
- Smiling at a neighbour when you usually feel too shy to do this.
- Phoning somebody when you feel lonely or need some help.
- Going for a walk with your baby.

Your examples from the last week or so, of compassionate behaviour that has helped you or others in the moment:

____

____

____

____

Examples of compassionate behaviour for the short term

- Looking for activities that you could do with your baby when your partner goes back to work.
- Looking for activities for yourself for when you feel ready to leave your baby with someone else.

- Taking your baby to spend an hour or so with people you will want your baby to get used to being looked after by.
- Cooking in larger quantities so there are meals for later in the week when you are more tired.
- Asking for help in caring and feeding your baby in the night so you can get more sleep.
- Looking for activities that you are excited to share with your baby and partner.

Your examples of compassionate behaviour for the short term

____

____

____

____

Examples of compassionate behaviour for the long term

- Being a secure base and safe haven for your baby – over and over again.
- Being responsive and kind to your baby when you are tired or cross.
- Addressing relationship difficulties with your partner.
- Learning to drive if this would help you and your family.
- Taking a course/learning new things.
- Teaching your baby things/providing them with new experiences.
- Sorting out moving house to a better environment for you and your family.
- Changing your diet to a healthier one.
- Seeking help for mental health/health issues when you have been used to not taking care of yourself.
- Seeking out opportunities to make new friends when you feel shy and uncertain of yourself.
- Trying to hold in mind and nurture old friends when you feel tired and have a lot to think about.
- Seeking help to improve your relationship with your baby when you are scared of people's reactions.
- Letting your partner develop a relationship with your baby when you fear your baby might end up loving them more than you.

- Standing up for yourself when you have felt unworthy or scared for years.
- Standing up for your child when you feel shy and scared.
- Taking care of yourself and your needs when you are used to putting others first.
- Saying no, and putting down boundaries with your child, from a place of compassion rather than anger or anxiety.
- Allowing people to help you.
- Joining the library for you and your baby.
- Remembering what you used to enjoy doing, and planning how to bring that back into your life again.

Your examples of compassionate behaviour in the long term

____

____

____

____

Courageous behaviour

Reading through the above lists, it is striking just how much courage many of these examples require. This is why courage is such an important aspect of compassionate behaviour. When we have a baby, things which we dismissed for ourselves might become things that we are determined to do for our baby. But they are often not easy. Indeed, we may have spent a large part of our lives struggling with them. You might notice yourself really digging in deep to find your courage, now you have had a baby. This is why the first part of changing from a pattern of threat to a pattern of compassion (the first 'stepping stone') is our posture – we first find a stable, grounded, steady 'dignified' posture, like a mountain or mighty oak tree – feeling our strength, courage, and commitment to doing this compassionate behaviour, even if we feel scared.

Our critic can often be close by, ready to dismiss what for us is a courageous act – 'What was so great about doing that? Everyone does that without even thinking about it?' This requires us to hold firm and strong in the face of our critic in order to remind ourselves (perhaps by revisiting your formulation) just why what we did was a big deal for us. We need our courageous and strong stance to stand up to the self-critic.

Parenting itself can be seen as a courageous act – we have no certainty as to how what we do now will impact our child in the long run – our children are perhaps our biggest experiment. So, we are trying as best we can to parent from our compassionate self, setting our child up in the best way we can, to help them flourish in life and be able to get through the inevitable tough times.

A misconception about compassion is that it is about being nice, or about love. These feelings may accompany compassionate acts, but they are not prerequisites and indeed don't need to be present at all. We might help a complete stranger who has fallen over in the street – and nothing about it feels like you are being nice or loving. Instead, you might be feeling a little scared yourself, concerned, anxious you might be making things worse, but still wanting to help somebody who is suffering. Indeed, mothers who are struggling with pre- or postnatal depression and feel numb, hopeless or panicky, some of whom feel no love at all for their baby, can still be astonishingly committed and motivated to helping their baby as best they can. It really is a monumental undertaking to maintain that focus despite being in high threat and without the feelings or hormonal systems in play that make this immensely difficult job of parenting so much easier. Here we really see how it is strength, commitment and courage that is core to compassion.

Sometimes compassionate behaviour may not seem nice at all; for example, not letting our child eat all the sweets they might want to, or encouraging ourselves to get on and do something that we are very anxious about but will help us in the long run, such as ringing up to sort out a payment that we missed, or arranging to talk to a teacher at our child's school about something we are unhappy about, when we are exceedingly unconfident and shy.

Looking back at our formulation, we discussed how we can get caught in tricky loops. This is where our ways of protecting ourselves (our safety strategies) cause unintended consequences which we then criticise ourselves for, triggering the very fears we were trying to protect ourselves from. Getting out of these loops means beginning to behave in new ways which fit with the life we want to begin to have, and the person we want to be. It is very hard and scary to do, as our fears can be strong, and our safety strategies may have been with us for our whole life. On top of that, we have brains that have evolved with 'better safe than sorry' strategies, so we tend to stick with what we know rather than risk trying something new and making things worse. So, we can see why trying new behaviour requires such strength, courage and commitment. But if we can manage this then the gains can be life changing.

Imagine you are a method actor who has been studying a particularly strong and courageous compassionate person or being for many months: how they move, how they sound if they speak, the expression on their face, how they interact with others. Now imagine stepping into this character and method acting 'as if' you are them. Notice how your body changes, notice your posture, how you move, how you sound, the expressions on your face, how you are in the world, how you interact with others.

How do you feel? What do you notice? What do you want to hold onto and remember from this?

____

____

____

____

From your formulation, what are some behaviours that you might want to start doing differently?

____

____

____

____

____

How might your compassionate mind help you try out a new behaviour?

____

____

____

____

____

For example:

- Honour the old safety strategy.
- Validate what you have gone through.
- Set in mind what is important to you about changing this behaviour – e.g. what might you really hope to do, or look forward to doing, that you struggle to do now? What would other people notice that you are doing differently? If you were looking at you in the future through your compassionate eyes, what would you see that is different? What might your child see is different?
- Tiny steps.
- How you (as this compassionate being) help yourself if the steps are too big.
- If you don't manage it this time – how you (as this compassionate being) help yourself with any disappointment and try again.
- Seeking help from others.
- Finding wisdom from yourself – how did you manage difficult things in the past? Times you have found more courage or strength than you imagined.
- Finding wisdom from others – health professionals, support groups, friends, family, books, courses, online.
- Taking in the achievement – letting it soak in.
- Being with your self-critic in a compassionate manner if it tries to dismiss what you did.

- Imagining the new behaviour before trying it – testing it out in imagination – seeing what you 'bump up against'.
- Writing new behaviour that you want to try on a postcard and carrying it with you, so that you are considering it more consciously as you go about your life.
- Trying it when it's easier, e.g. talking to friends or your partner and testing with them.
- Thinking it first.
- Or just holding it as a new part of you – no need to act yet.
- Making tiny changes in responses to others.

Reflections and notes: What would you like to take hold of and remember from this section on compassionate behaviour? What would you like to take forward and try? What might be your next steps?

___

___

___

___

Section 7:

Working with our difficulties using our compassionate mind

Module 44: Our fears, blocks and resistances to the three flows of compassion

To manage the inevitable struggles and suffering that are part of our lives as humans, we need to be able to access all three flows of compassion. That is, being able to ask for and take in compassion from others, giving compassion to others and giving compassion to ourselves (and also allowing in the compassion we give to ourselves).

Think of the three flows of compassion – compassion flowing from us to others, flowing from ourselves into ourselves, and flowing from others into us. If you put them in a ladder of hardest to easiest, which flow would be hardest for you, and which the easiest?

My ladder:

1. Hardest flow of compassion ⇧ ____________________
2. The one in the middle ⇧ ____________________
3. Easiest flow of compassion ⇧ ____________________

As humans we generally stick to whatever is the easiest and avoid the hardest, but for us to feel safe and to be able to flourish, we need to be able to access all three flows.

This is also what we would want for our child – **after all, would there be one or more of these flows that we would suggest our child should avoid? What might their life be like if they did?**

____

____

____

____

____

We don't start off struggling with any of these flows of compassion – these struggles come from our experiences, perhaps entwined with our genes, our particular brain, set-up, our personality and so on – so in other words – not our fault. However, we can see the impact it might have if our baby didn't have one or more of the flows available to them, and this can help to really understand the impact on us too.

Exercise: Looking at the flow of compassion that you rated as the hardest for you

1. What are the benefits for you in *not* engaging with this flow of compassion?

____

____

____

____

____

2. What might you gain if you *could* engage with this flow of compassion?

____

____

____

____

____

As with any behaviour we find difficult, and as we would when helping our child with difficult things too, we start at the bottom of the ladder of difficultly at the point where it is challenging but not too difficult.

Which flow would this be for you?

____

____

Rather than jumping sections to the one that you are wanting to work on, or the one you feel is the hardest for you, have a read through all three flows. Sometimes we can be surprised when we really start to engage with each one. We may then wish to re-order our ladder of easiest to hardest.

Reflections and notes: What would you like to take hold of and remember from this section on fears, blocks and resistance to the three flows of compassion? What would you like to take forward and try? What might be your next steps?

____

____

____

____

Module 45: Compassion to others

Some of the fears, blocks or resistances that people experience with this flow are things like:

- 'If I show any compassion towards that person, then they will want more help from me than I can give them at the moment.'
- 'They will just take advantage of me and use me.'
- 'They will think I am foolish and laugh at me, or think I consider myself above them and then get cross with me.'
- 'I will end up giving compassion out, but no-one will give any back.'

My fears of showing compassion to others are:

____

____

____

____

What are some specific things that you would like to be able to do if you could become comfortable with this particular flow of compassion?

____

____

____

____

e.g. 'I would like to connect more with my baby. Especially when he cries. At the moment my fear shuts me down, and I become a bit cold and cross with him.'

Why is this important to you?

---

e.g. 'Because I know that this isn't the kind of mother I want to be, and I really would hate to be treated this way by my mother when I was upset.'

How would you like to be instead?

---

e.g. 'I would like to want to pick him up when he is upset and hold him close and settle him. This would make him feel safe and let him know that I am here for him.'

What gets in the way of being this version of yourself? For example, when he cries, what version of you pops up instead?

---

e.g. 'When he cries, there is an anxious part of me that pops up and puts my stomach in knots. I want the crying to stop. Then this angry part seems to swoop in to save the anxious part and says in my head to the baby "What is the matter with you? Why are you crying over that? Your mother is doing everything she can for you. Just give her a break, you demanding, ungrateful thing!" I don't want to say that to my baby, so I just go cold and quiet, but I don't want to pick him up.'

How might your compassionate self or other help you to understand where your current struggles with this have come from? E.g. Can you remember that anxious or angry response to the cries of you or others in your past? How were you responded to when you cried?

____

____

____

____

How did you need others to respond to you when you were upset?

____

____

____

____

How might your compassionate self or other help you to begin to be the way you would like to be now? (The step-by-step process of trying out behavioural change as used in the assertiveness section later in the book may help here.)

____

____

____

____

For example:

- Connect with memories of when you have been able to send compassion to others.
- Practise sending this out when it's easier, e.g. to strangers you drive or walk past, or to people you imagine in their houses. Perhaps practise with some set words, e.g. 'May you be well. May you be happy. May you find peace.'
- Practise gratitude: perhaps just making a note each day of three things that you are grateful for (different ones each day).
- Imagine all the people that have been involved in bringing you something that you like, e.g. your favourite cup, including the potter, the people that dug up the clay and made the porcelain for the cup, the person that designed the packaging and the one that made it, the shop worker . . . and send out a warm thank you to them all.
- As you walk around, imagine sending out your compassion secretly like a warm ray of light or mist.
- Test out tiny compassionate acts or gestures and see how it feels to do them. Notice whether any of your fears come true. If so, how does your compassionate self help you manage them?
- Notice what your heartfelt wish might be for particular people from your strong, wise, caring compassionate mind, even if you don't feel able to express it or let them know.
- Write a compassionate letter to them, even if you never post it.
- Write some compassionate words or a message on a postcard to a person you struggle to show compassion to and just carry it in your pocket, seeing how it feels to have it with you.
- Become aware of how your compassionate self or other might help you be assertive and clear about what you can and can't offer if you feel you may be taken advantage of.
- Notice how your compassionate self or other might help you if you get ridiculed or shamed for trying to be helpful and compassionate or if you misjudge it or carry it out a bit clumsily.
- How might your compassionate self or other help you if your compassion to someone else was rebuffed or rejected (perhaps because they have a fear of compassion from others), as it is hard to be rebuffed after plucking up the courage to send compassion out.

Imagine you are a method actor who has been studying a person who finds it easy to be compassionate to others for many months: how they move, how they sound if they speak, the expression on their face, how they interact with others. Now imagine stepping into this character and method acting as if you are them. Notice how your body changes, notice your posture, how you move, how you sound, the expressions on your face, how you are in the world, how you interact with others.

How do you feel? What do you notice? What do you want to hold onto and remember from this?

____

____

____

____

____

Reflections and notes: What would you like to take hold of and remember from this section on compassion to others? What would you like to take forward and try? What might be your next steps?

____

____

____

____

Module 46: Giving and accepting self-compassion

Common fears, blocks and resistances to being self-compassionate include:

- 'I will let myself off the hook and become lazy or not try.'
- 'If I am compassionate to myself then others might feel that they don't need to make the effort to be compassionate to me.'
- 'People might think that I am being self-indulgent and selfish.'
- 'I might forget about my baby if I focus on myself.'
- 'I will realise how sad or how angry I feel and then these would get out of control.'

What are some of your fears of being self-compassionate?

____

____

____

____

____

What might it be like for your child as they grew up, if their ability to be self-compassionate was, for some reason, lost or didn't work?

____

____

____

____

____

Why might you want your child to be able to be self-compassionate as they grow up?

What might be helpful to you about being self-compassionate?

Why might your child wish that you could become self-compassionate? What might their hopes be for you if you could become self-compassionate?

How might your compassionate other/image understand your struggles with being self-compassionate? How might they validate you?

What does your compassionate other understand about your struggles from their wise mind? For example, from their understanding of your experiences, your genes, the environment you grew up in – none of which you chose?

What might its heartfelt wish be for you? Why might it deeply wish you could bring compassion to yourself?

How might it help you to start on your journey to self-compassion?

E.g. Tiny step by tiny step

Imagine a part of you that is struggling, or that you struggle with, were to appear in front of you, sitting on a chair? Imagine relating to it as if it were a beloved person, child, animal or object. How would you be with it? What might you say to it? How might you help it? What might your heartfelt wish be for it?

Bring compassion to parts of your body, e.g. your womb that carried your baby, your hand that has done so many things for you over all these years, your eyes that allow you to see your child and the beauty in the world. What would you say to these parts of you? What would you wish for them? How might you be with them?

Bring a gentle touch and care to your hand. Perhaps apply some moisturiser. Imagine your skin expressing its gratitude to you, that you have noticed it and given it some care.

How did that feel? What was that like?

Prepare some food or a drink for yourself with the same care that you prepare food, or drink, or a breastfeed, for your baby.

How was that? What might you want to remember from that?

Prepare a space that is important to you with the same care you prepared your baby's space before their arrival. Perhaps making the place where you feed your baby as comfortable and pleasurable for you as possible, or your bed, an area in your house or your garden, even if it is no bigger than a seat.

Which space would you like to prepare? What would you like to do to make it as comfortable and pleasurable for you as possible?

____

____

____

____

____

As the feelings of self-compassion become more familiar, make a list of areas that are more challenging e.g. particular emotions you find hard, behaviours you'd like to change in yourself, things you'd like to achieve but feel stuck with, relationships you find tricky.

My list of areas that could benefit from my self-compassion:

____

____

____

____

____

Order them from easiest to hardest:

Easiest: ____

____

____

____

Hardest: ____

Pick the easiest and then from your wise, warm, caring, strong, courageous, compassionate mind, brainstorm ways in which you might set about helping yourself with this. Perhaps ask others for their suggestions and their help too. How might you help your child if they came to you with this?

Imagine 'If I were compassionate to myself, what words might I write on this postcard to myself?' Carry this postcard around in your pocket and see how it feels to have it with you.

What might you write on your postcard?

Write a letter to yourself from your compassionate other:

Imagine you are a method actor, and you have been studying your compassionate other/image or a compassionate figure from, say, a children's television series, film or book. You have been studying them for months – how they walk, what they wear, the way they move, the sound of their voice, how they interact with people. Imagine stepping into their body and moving around the room – how would you be towards *you* if that character were to come across you? What might you say with your warm, kind voice? What might you understand with your wise mind? How might your courage and strength play out? If you were to swap back into your own body, how might it feel to have that compassionate character with you? How might it feel to have them in your life, helping you, guiding you, supporting you, encouraging you, just being with you as a warm, dependable presence? How might you be?

____

____

____

____

____

____

____

____

____

____

____

____

____

____

____

How do you feel? What do you notice? What do you want to hold onto and remember from this?

Imagine you are a method actor who has been studying a person who has finally become comfortable at being self-compassionate, for many months: how they move, how they sound if they speak, the expression on their face, how they interact with others, how they interact with themselves. Now imagine stepping into this character and method acting 'as if' you are them. Notice how your body changes, your posture, how you move, how you sound, the expressions on your face, how you are in the world, how you interact with others, how you interact with yourself.

How do you feel? What do you notice? What do you want to hold onto and remember from this?

Reflections and notes: What would you like to take hold of and remember from this section on working with the difficulties of self-compassion? What would you like to take forward and try? What might be your next steps?

___

___

___

___

Module 47: Seeking and accepting help and compassion from others

People often say that self-compassion is the flow that they find hardest, but when looking more closely, many people's greatest struggle is in fact with receiving compassion from others. This can be particularly so for women brought up in societies where girls and women are expected to be giving, self-sacrificing, and caring of others rather than receiving care themselves. Receiving care then becomes an unknown, not part of your sense of self, and shamed or frowned upon. There can also be a great vulnerability in opening oneself to receiving care because of the degree of trust required; that the other person will help you rather than taking advantage of you.

Common fears, blocks and resistances to receiving compassion include:

- 'If I let someone care for me, then I will owe them help in return, and I just don't feel I have enough resources for myself, let alone for others.'
- 'Rather than helping me, they may take advantage of me.'
- 'They may be just helping me out of pity, rather than genuine compassion.'
- 'If I let compassion in, I will collapse and crumble into sadness, then I will not be able to look after my children.'
- 'I would feel small and childlike, like I am sitting being held by a big, kind grown-up. Even though that's what I crave, I need to be the grown-up myself for my baby.'
- 'I don't feel worthy of care and compassion from others.'

So even though women in some societies are shaped to give rather than receive care, when it comes to the perinatal period, we have evolved to share care of our babies. So, we can have two opposing pulls – to give care to others (and now as a mother, there are additional expectations that we will be all-giving and caring), and on the opposite side – to have care *from* others for ourselves, and for our baby.

In many societies, a baby is viewed as a valuable and precious new member of the 'tribe' or group. The mother would be regarded as precious too and looked after accordingly. There would be many people clamouring to care for the baby and in some societies the baby would have around ten 'alloparents' (people who regularly care for them). Imagine having all these people who are desperate to look after your baby, rather than feeling you have to ask a favour.

And the dynamics of giving and receiving 'favours' is also something that seems to be part of our evolutionary make-up. There is evidence that, like us, other Great Apes also track whether they are in debt to others in terms of favours, or in credit.

Do you prefer to be in debt or in credit to others when it comes to favours? Why?

____

____

____

____

____

How do you manage this? (e.g. never asking for help so are never in debt, not worrying too much about it, it will all even out in the end, keeping a mental note and feeling relieved when a chance comes to help someone in return.)

____

____

____

____

____

This can be a real issue for new mothers who do not have ready access to help, particularly the kind of help that they don't feel the need to pay back – such as from their own mothers. People may say, 'Don't forget to ask if you need any help' or 'Get somebody to have your baby as you need time to yourself', not really appreciating the hurdles that would need to be overcome to do this. This results in the sadly all too common experience of many women trying to manage their baby entirely on their own.

Added to all of this might be experiences where we have been taken advantage of, shamed, or psychologically or physically 'left' when we were hoping for compassion from others. This makes the whole issue of seeking and receiving compassion now we have had a baby like climbing an impossibly high mountain, at a time when we are particularly depleted.

However, research is beginning to show that receiving compassion from others may actually be the most important of the three flows in terms of our wellbeing, as it seems to have a particularly strong buffering effect in all sorts of challenging circumstances. And of course, this is the 'original' flow of compassion if you like – when we are born we do not give compassion to others, or to ourselves. Instead, we are utterly dependent on the care-giving and compassion of others for our very survival. We are wired from the very beginning of our existence to require care and compassion to survive, to learn and to flourish. That wiring never leaves us or diminishes.

Therefore, despite the mountain of difficulties, we need compassion, care and support from others, particularly when we are pregnant and have a new baby.

So how might our compassionate self or compassionate other/image help us with this?

Imagine stepping in to that compassionate part of you, or stepping into a compassionate character from television, films, stories or real life and pretend that you are them for a little while. Feel your body become upright, steady and stable ('dignified' posture, body like a mountain or an ancient, mighty tree). Slow down your in and your out breath. Allow your breathing to become slow, smooth and rhythmic. Bring your warm, kind face, and warm, kind voice to this practice – perhaps greeting yourself, or your breath, with joy and warmth. Connect with your intention to be as caring and helpful as you can. Connect with the wisdom you have gained across the whole of your life – about yourself, and about others too. Connect with your strength and your courage.

Now imagine coming across that part of you that struggles to ask for help from others, and/or struggles to take that help and compassion into yourself. How would your compassionate self be with that part? How would it feel towards it? What might it say to it? What might its heartfelt wish for that part be? How would it work to help that part?

Some suggestions:

- If we struggle to receive help and care from others it can be easier to engage with compassionate self rather than compassionate other (but work towards engaging with compassionate other – this could be your most needed and helpful practice).
- Validate that we need it, but that it can be so hard to ask for or allow for many reasons, none of which are our fault, despite how easily people offer it.
- Carry with you your written intention on a postcard to notice and consider compassion to yourself – nothing to do but notice.

What would you write on your postcard?

- Run through in your imagination what it might be like to receive compassion. Notice areas of tension and resistance, see if you can capture these in words, drawings or paintings – this can help your compassionate part begin to understand the fears, blocks and resistances, what it needs to help you with.

What might it be like for me to receive compassion? My areas of tension and resistance?

____

____

____

____

____

Notice other people receiving compassion – perhaps from you, perhaps from others – how do they receive it? What does receiving compassion look like? Perhaps notice in your baby – how do they receive your care, help and compassion?

____

____

____

____

____

- Practise resisting 'brushing off' kindness and compassion – perhaps accepting with a warm 'thank you' and see how that feels.

How did that feel?

____

____

- Practise the feeling of *allowing*, of allowing in compassion from others, starting with the easy, e.g. allowing in a smile from someone else, the moving out of the way for you and your buggy, the offer of making you a cup of tea. Become familiar with the sensation and process of allowing, in a gentle, tiny step by tiny step manner – no rush.

List here what you are practising allowing, or have practised:

How is it feeling? What are you noticing?

Notice with your baby – what does allowing look like from their point of view?

If part of the block is a fear of getting into a 'compassion debt' where you now owe more than you can currently give – how might your compassionate self or compassionate other be with you, and help you with this fear?

How would you help your child to receive compassion from others? How would you help your child to ask for help as they grow up?

How would you help a good friend to seek support?

How would you help a good friend to take in that compassion?

How would you help your good friend or your child deal with the rejection of their request for help?

How would your compassionate self or compassionate other help you if your courageous reaching out and asking for help was dismissed or rejected?

How would your compassionate self or other help you to manage reaching out again for help in the future after that setback?

- Practise experiencing and expressing gratitude at the offer of care and compassion towards yourself even if at the moment, for whatever reason, you cannot take it in (sometimes in our panic to defend ourselves from compassion, our threat system makes us forget to appreciate the kind intention of others even if we cannot accept it – but we can practise remembering it – even if it comes after the event).

How does that feel? What do you notice?

- Know that in the scheme of things you will be offering your compassionate self when you can, even if it is years down the line.

When can you imagine you might be offering your compassionate self to others in the future (this may be in many years)?

- Try a smile and a sending out of compassionate intentions, light, mist even if you can't offer anything more than that at the moment – that in itself makes a difference (imagine how it feels when someone gives you a genuinely warm, understanding smile).

How does that feel? What do you notice?

- Connect with others in a similar position where the challenges of giving and receiving care are understood, e.g. parent and baby groups, online meet-ups, breastfeeding support, where it may be easier to help in that moment, e.g. minding a sleeping baby while its mum quickly goes to the toilet.

Who might be possible people? Who is there in your life at the moment where it does feel OK to give little moments of help and compassion to?

* Receiving a gift from others – allowing others to give you a gift and to give it to you freely without any need for it to be repaid, is a gift that we can give to others. Think about how it feels when you wish to give something freely, just to be kind, just to be helpful, with no expectation of repayment. Notice how it feels to be able to do that for your baby – to give them care with grace and delight, expecting nothing in return, just enjoying the act of giving that gift. Now imagine practising receiving the gift with gratitude and delight and letting the feeling of needing to repay it be acknowledged and then allowed to disappear.

How does that feel? How might your compassionate mind help you with this?

Imagine you are a method actor who has been studying (for many months) a person who can seek and receive compassion and help from others: how they move, how they sound if they speak, the expression on their face, how they interact with others. Now imagine stepping into this character and method acting 'as if' you are them. Notice how your body changes, your posture, how you move, how you sound, the expressions on your face, how you are in the world, how you interact with others.

How do you feel? What do you notice? What do want to hold onto and remember from this?

Reflections and notes: What would you like to take hold of and remember from this section on working with difficulties of seeking and accepting help and compassion from others? What would you like to take forward and try? What might be your next steps?

Module 48: When we feel unworthy of compassion from others or from ourselves

This is a big and painful area and one which is the focus of a great deal of therapeutic work. Indeed, it is this very issue that inspired Professor Paul Gilbert to develop compassion-focused therapy (CFT) and the compassionate mind approach, after many years of clinical work and research with the most desperate of patients. And this is why many therapists working with, and people suffering with, this particular issue, are turning to CFT. It can be hard to navigate this on your own and you may wish to seek a therapist to help you with it.

It may be that you skip this module until you have someone who can work with you, or you skim read it as if 'from a distance' or just touch it lightly. But it is such an important area that it can be helpful to have at least a sense of how you might go about working with, and taking care, of this very sore and tender part, when you feel ready to. After all, these experiences and beliefs prevent us from accessing two out of the three flows of compassion (compassion from others, and self-compassion), two such important flows for our wellbeing, particularly during the perinatal period.

These fears and beliefs can be behind a struggle to allow our baby to love us, as we feel undeserving of their love, and fear that one day they will discover how bad we really are and then reject us. In fact, this can be a belief that is held about anybody – that *'you only like/ love/ care for me, because you have not yet discovered how awful I really am'*. This makes asking for, and allowing in, the care and compassion that we are wired to need when we have a new baby feel so utterly impossible. We may have managed to navigate through life by not letting people get too close to us, or by choosing a partner who struggles to give compassion and care. But having a baby can be a time when these safety strategies are stretched and tested and may no longer work. Or when our need for help and care becomes far greater than ever before, because of evolutionary mechanisms that swing into action, such as our need for our mother (or an ideal of a mother), and our need to share the care of our baby.

So how might we approach this issue? As ever, we need the best elements of compassion that we can muster – which of course may be tricky when two of the three flows of compassion feel fraught with fears, blocks and resistances. But there are many elements still available to us. We just need to go step by step, building slowly. Even if it is a life's work. Because this is so important – imagine a precious child who has had to have a feeding tube and needs to learn to eat normally again, or one who has had a damaged leg and needs to learn to walk again, or a foster child who has been so scared to love that they shut down – we wouldn't just give up, or assume there is no point trying. They need these areas in order to live well, so we would keep persisting for as long as it takes – still trying, still facing in that direction, even if it takes our whole lifetime – just helping them, tiny bit by tiny bit. And that is the same for us.

- Firstly, as with anything we are approaching that is difficult, we need our steadiness, strength and stability. So, find your steady posture – body like a mountain, or mighty tree – sitting or walking, whatever allows you to best feel the strength and steadiness of your body. Slow your in and your out breath, and bring that kind, warm face and voice to this.

Get in touch with your motivation for doing this – what you would like to be able to do or feel as a consequence of working on receiving compassion and love from others and from yourself? Why does it feel important to tackle this difficult area?

___

___

___

___

___

It may not be clear; just that you know in some way that you need it is enough. Step into that part of you that can be deeply caring. And tap into the wisdom you have acquired about yourself and others through the course of your life. Find that part of you that has courage, more courage than you perhaps have imagined – the part of you that has strength to keep doing difficult things, even when they are scary. Just notice what it feels like to be filled with this, to move around, or to imagine moving around. Perhaps imagine being in your compassionate place as you work on this – a place where you feel free and at ease and can be just as you need to be.

How does this feel to be inhabiting this part? Anything you want to note and remember from this practice?

____

____

____

____

____

Imagine you are a method actor who has been studying a compassionate person or being for many months: how they move, how they sound if they speak, the expression on their face, how they interact with others, particularly critical people. Now imagine stepping into this character and imagine method acting 'as if' you are them. Notice how your body changes, your posture, how you move, how you sound, the expressions on your face, how you are in the world.

How would this compassionate character be with the critic and the person being criticised?

____

____

____

____

____

How do you feel? What do you notice? What do you want to hold onto and remember from this?

____

____

____

As this compassionate character, meet with yourself and validate yourself for the suffering you have experienced through your life because of this struggle, and the courage and strength you have in even having a go with this.

What might you say to yourself? How might you be with yourself? Perhaps write yourself a compassionate letter, postcard or some compassionate words.

- From your compassionate mind, turn towards the origins of these fears of being unlovable, unworthy and undeserving of compassion. (Just do whatever feels right to you with this section. It may be something for another time, or something you just skim read.) Perhaps revisit your formulation or draw out your formulation in order to understand what happened in your life, the fears that these experiences created about yourself and about others, the safety strategies you developed consciously or unconsciously to try to prevent the fears happening again, and then the unintended consequences of these safety strategies. Perhaps imagine just watching with compassion, from a distance, a speeded-up film of your parents' lives, your life in your mother's belly, your birth, your childhood, your teenage years, all the way to your current life.

What do you see? (This is not about blame, but just about observation, curiosity and discovery – a process of trying to understand and shed light on all this.)

You might notice for example that, just like your baby, no child is born bad, unworthy, or undeserving of love, care and compassion. In fact, the opposite – they depend on this for life – they cannot live without somebody else caring for them. So, at some point a child begins to learn or feel that they are unlovable or 'bad'. This occurs through the experiences that happen to them that may create a bodily collection of feelings that we label as 'bad'. These feelings may be accompanied by a sense from others that we have done something wrong. Perhaps we are told this explicitly, or we pick this up from subtle cues such as the way somebody turns away from us or looks at us. We associate these horrible feelings, this sense of *feeling* bad, with a sense that we *are* bad. Both aspects come from outside of us. They are nothing to do with us. If we had been taken at birth and put in a loving family, we are unlikely to be feeling this way – it is not our fault. We just *feel* it is. Because we are too young and too vulnerable to understand this, or to argue back, this feeling lodges in us, often for life. But it doesn't need to. As we begin to understand why it's come to be within us, and we begin to work with it with care, courage, and tenderness, it begins to dissolve and disappear.

To understand this more deeply – how might you set about trying to create a child that feels bad, unworthy, unlovable?

How might you instead go about trying to create a child that feels lovable and worthy of love and compassion?

____

____

____

____

____

- This is likely to bring up lots of emotions. Keep anchored with your steady body like a mountain or mighty tree, breathe into the feelings, and around the feelings, so there is a sense that there is space for them. Allow yourself to connect with the emotions lightly with a gentle touch, from a distance, with a steady, compassionate mind. Or perhaps imagine sitting with or holding the emotions, like you would a dear child who is experiencing these emotions – nothing to do but be with them, from your strong, steady, caring, wise, compassionate mind.

What was this like to do? How might your compassionate mind be helping you with this? What might you want to take note of and remember from this?

____

____

____

____

____

- Imagine that this feeling bad, or unworthy or unlovable could appear, sitting in a chair.

From your steady, caring, wise, strong, courageous, compassionate mind, how might you be with it? What might you say to it if you were to speak to it? What might your heartfelt wish or wishes for it be? How might you set about trying to help it over time?

____

____

____

____

____

- Imagine now that for a moment you could swap into the body of that part that feels bad, or unworthy or unlovable, and you look out and see this strong, wise, steady, warm, compassionate mind here with you.

What is it like to know it is here to help you, as long as it takes, for your whole life? It is not going to leave you. That it understands you inside and out. That there is nothing you need to confess or reveal to it – it knows you completely and understands and accepts you. It knows just how hard this is for you. It is here to help you, slowly, steadily, step by step.

How does this feel to have this part with you? How does your body feel?

____

____

____

____

____

- Now imagine swapping back into your compassionate mind and body – feeling your strength and steadiness – body like a mountain or mighty tree, slowing down your breathing, bringing your warm, kind face and voice to this. Finding that wise, strong, courageous, caring part of you again. Noticing how it feels to be back in this part.

Notice how it feels that you are able to approach and be with this struggling part that feels bad and unworthy in this way.

What was this like? What did you notice? What would you like to take note of and remember?

____

____

____

____

____

Imagine you are a method actor who has been studying (for many months) a person or being (perhaps an animal or pet) who feels worthy of love and compassion: how they move, how they sound if they speak, the expression on their face, how they interact with others. Now imagine stepping into this character and imagine method acting 'as if' you are them. Notice how your body changes, your posture, how you move, how you sound, the expressions on your face, how you are in the world, how you interact with others.

How do you feel? What do you notice? What do you want to hold onto and remember from this?

____

____

____

____

____

Working with this over time:

- Work gently and slowly, like you would with an animal that has had a difficult early life or has been harmed or hurt – gently, slowly, knowing it will take time, but you are here for the long term, building trust, never letting them down, working with gentleness, kindness, but persistence – you know this is worth sticking with for them.
- Work with the end fear – sometimes we cannot begin work, because we aren't confident we could deal with the 'what if's', no matter how unlikely they might be. There is no point people trying to reassure us that 'that won't happen', or 'you'll be fine'. You need to know yourself that you will manage even the most feared of things – and this is what compassion is all about. When there is no way out, when the worst *is* happening, we have a part of us with us, that is helping us to bear and get through even this.

So, a 'what if' here might be 'What if I do let people love me and give me compassion and then they *do* reject me?' This is a possibility – people may fall out of love with us, or move on from us, even when we are at our best – after all, we may not find we fit with many others in the world even when they are at their best – it is not their fault, or our fault, it is just the nature of having a diverse range of people in the world. So how do we bear rejection – after all, that is our most profound fear – but then get back up and reach out again? Because we still function at our best as humans when connected to others.

We will need this when our children reject us, as they are very likely to do, particularly as this is also a 'job' or 'task' of adolescence – for a child to find a way of detaching from their parents so they can move away and find a mate, like all animals must do. But this will also happen when your child is younger and they 'hate you' or 'wish you weren't my mother!' as you work your way through this balance of letting them learn and grow and keeping them steady and safe.

How would you help your child develop the ability to get back up from rejection, recover, and be able to reach out again? (This is a painful but unavoidable part of human life and this is why we need compassion – normal human life is full of both suffering and joy.)

___

___

___

How might your compassionate self help you if a rejection were to happen? It can help to write this out as a compassionate letter or list or plan, a kind of 'This is what we will do if this were to happen – it will feel awful, but we will get you back up and you will be OK. We will get through it together.'

Reflections and notes: What would you like to take hold of and remember from this section on working with feeling unworthy of compassion from ourselves or others? What would you like to take forward and try? What might be your next steps?

Module 49: When the person who make us feel unworthy is someone we rely on or live with

We may still have in our life the person or people who are the source of our sense of feeling unlovable and unworthy. Even if we have broken contact with family members with whom we have a difficult relationship, once we have a baby we can be drawn back to them because of old, evolved mechanisms of needing to share the care of our baby. Particularly so to our mother, even if she is not really the kind of mother we would wish for. This is very tricky because we need their help, but their manner towards us is not helpful – back to the similar trap we experienced as a child. However, we are not children anymore, even though most people feel like they are children again when in the presence of their parents (our conditioned ways of relating, as children, and as parents, are incredibly strong). This is where our compassionate mind training is so helpful. We can practise being at our compassionate best and most compassionately assertive, in order to set in motion different ways of relating (see section on assertiveness). This helps us in not coming from a position of blame, but one of 'It is not your fault, but it is your responsibility'.

How might your compassionate mind help you with this? (Switch into your compassionate mind first before you answer this – 'Body like a mountain, breath like the wind, mind like the blue sky', warm, kind face and voice. Stepping into the part of you that has great wisdom, strength, courage and a deep commitment to being as helpful and caring as you can.)

____

____

____

____

With this work it may become clearer and clearer that the person you live with and depend on, who may be the father or mother of your baby, is also the source of your self-criticism and of feeling unworthy. You really may need to turn to others to help you with this, particularly if you are scared of them. Your safety and the safety of your baby is the most important thing. This can be a very entangled situation where you may financially depend on them, may have become so beaten down that you do not imagine you can live without them or find somebody else who would love and take care of you. You may feel that your child having their parent in their lives is more important than your wellbeing.

Again, as ever, changing this situation is probably going to begin with a light touch, with a turning towards yourself in a different manner, with a beginning to disentangle this in your mind, perhaps with the help of others, with a bringing of your compassionate mind to this.

What advice would you give a friend or your grown-up child in this situation? How might your compassionate mind help you with this?

____

____

____

____

What might be your first steps with this?

____

____

____

____

Examples of first steps:

- Just holding in your mind, a wish and a commitment for this to be different.

- Carrying this wish round with you, perhaps represented by a pebble or picture you carry in your pocket or a bracelet or piece of jewellery you wear.
- Becoming clearer what it is your compassionate mind would like for you and your baby in the future (not the practicalities of how to get there – as these can throw us into our threat. Having a clear vision of why we are engaging with such a difficult thing helps us to take the steps to eventually get there and keeps a focus on why we are making these changes, especially when things get hard).
- Bringing your compassionate mind to the person that is harmful – very hard to do – and not to 'let them off the hook' or to disarm yourself, but to disentangle yourself from needing to be the solution to, or protecting them from, whatever causes them to act in this way. Finding, if we can, a genuine wish that they too can find what they need to be able to live a life free of having to be this way.
- Finding other people who you can begin to talk this over with; friends, family members, organisations who specifically help with this area, a counsellor/therapist, health visitor or GP.

Reflections and notes: What would you like to take hold of and remember from this section on working with the difficulty of when the person who makes us feel unworthy is someone we rely on or live with? What would you like to take forward and try? What might be your next steps?

____

____

____

____

Module 50: When the 'person' who makes us feel unworthy is our internal self-critic

(See also section on working with our inner critic for more in-depth work.)

The source of what is making us feel 'bad' about ourselves may be a part of ourselves. We may carry our experiences and memories with us of feeling unlovable and unworthy of care and compassion. Our self-critic can be a constant everyday (and night) stimulus of these feelings within us. In the section on working on our critic we looked at how our self-critic can develop, and the functions it may have. It can serve as a kind of safety strategy in that it may trigger us into a submissive 'one-down' position when it criticises us, which we may have learned was safer than being angry or challenging, or even lively and self-confident. It may serve to keep us feeling unworthy as a way of preventing us from assuming we are worthy of love and care, then reaching out to somebody, but then being met by rejection and humiliation. Or that without our self-critic we might stand up taller, and a little more confidently, and then get unwanted attention or hurt in some way.

However, the self-critic may not have come about as a safety strategy but instead could be an internalised voice of an actual critic from our lives. In a practice where people are invited to imagine watching their critic interacting with them as if watching a play that is far away on a stage, sometimes people will suddenly recognise that the words and manner of their critic are those of a real person such as a parent. Without realising it, they had been carrying that person inside of them for all of these years. So, it can be no wonder we remain feeling unworthy and unlovable when we are still being told this repeatedly by our self-critic.

How might your compassionate self help you with this internalised critic?

Switch into your compassionate mind first before you answer this – 'Body like a mountain, breath like the wind, mind like the blue sky,' warm, kind face and voice. Stepping into the part of you that has great wisdom, strength, courage and a deep commitment to being as helpful and caring as you can. Remember, as you get your compassionate mind,

that your strong dignified posture, your strength and your courage are crucial starting points when facing your critic. Your motivation to be helpful not harmful, and your wisdom are also important.

Sometimes just knowing where our inner critic has come from can be enough.

Where might it have come from for you?

Imagine looking back at your life as if looking down from a mountain onto your early/earlier experiences, or from a cloud or other high place where you can observe safely from a distance with steady curiosity. Imagine your life rolling backwards like watching a film backwards at fast speed. It can be very enlightening to watch the film further back to include you in your mother's womb and then further back to your parents' lives and early lives too.

The internal critical voice can have become a habit; a reflexive way of being with and responding to ourselves, as it has been with us as such an intrinsic, regular part of our lives.

We can then work with it like any habit we are trying to break. It is of course a very tough one to break, but like any habit still entirely possible.

> *Rather than continuing to feed a habit of self-criticism, we are creating a new habit; that of compassionate responding.*

How might your compassionate mind set about helping you to break this habit?

How might you help your child break a habit, for example when potty training, moving from a cot into their own 'big bed', or moving from a sipper cup to a proper cup?

What might you take from this to help you with your internal self-critic?

Some ideas that might help:

- At first it can be enough just to notice this voice or part with curiosity – 'Ah, so this is when it comes up. And then this is what happens within me when it does.' Nothing to do but observe and discover.
- We could map out or draw out the process of what happens to trigger the critic, how the critic reacts, then the impact of that. This visual representation can make clearer the precise function of the critic. It also enables the playing around with what might happen if a different part of us were to come in at that point instead of the critic.
- We could imagine we are watching a play from a distance that has been videoed, then watch it back frame by frame (we can change the colour, make it black and white, turn down the volume or make it go faster or slower) just to learn the process that occurs when the words of the critic get triggered and our body and mind then respond. This helps to give some separation from it.
- Then over time we can experiment with acting in a slightly different way, for example just letting the critical words run their course as if we are letting a bath empty, or practising not quite listening to the words as if they are an annoying fly buzzing somewhere in the room. We are beginning to break the association.
- Some people suggest shouting at the critic or telling it to go away or shut up. However, this may just stimulate our own threat system. This can be experimented with to see what happens.

What do you imagine might happen if you shouted at your inner critic, or told it to go away or shut up?

____

____

____

____

We can compare this to trying to respond to this from our compassionate mind, so with confidence, steadiness, non-blame, wisdom and curiosity. Here we are noticing what normally triggers our self-critic, then responding instead with our compassionate mind. We are loosening the link between the trigger (e.g. a negative comment from a parent about our parenting of our baby) and our self-critic, but then beginning to replace the self-critic with our compassionate mind. We are now creating a new habit, the habit of compassionate responding.

What do you imagine might happen if you responded to your critic with your compassionate mind?

(Remember to switch into your compassionate mind first before considering this:

'Body like a mountain, breath like the wind, mind like the blue sky', warm, kind face and voice. Stepping into the part of you that has great wisdom, strength, courage and a deep commitment to being as helpful and caring as you can.)

____

____

____

____

So how might our compassionate mind respond to a negative comment from a parent about our parenting?

(Remember the oxygen mask principle: the compassionate mind will respond to us first and then the other person, e.g. validating us first so we 'switch systems' and then can respond to the other person from this different pattern that the switching into the different pattern of our compassionate mind now gives us.)

____

____

____

____

Exercise: Stepping into the role of a compassionate other and meeting with our critic

Imagine you are a method actor who has been studying a compassionate person or being for many months: how they move, how they sound if they speak, the expression on their face, how they interact with others, particularly critical people. Now imagine stepping into this character and imagine method acting 'as if' you are them. Notice how your body changes, your posture, how you move, how you sound, the expressions on your face, how you are in the world, how you interact with the critic and the person being criticised.

How do you feel? What do you notice? What do you want to hold onto and remember from this?

____

____

____

____

Here we are replacing the self-critical habitual response with a new one. If our self-critic still feels strong and present then we can imagine our compassionate mind, or a strong, steady compassionate other/being arriving and being with the critic. Just bringing their strong, wise, understanding compassionate mind to understand the fear that drives the self-critic, or the experiences that created that self-critic that were not their fault. But then still responding to the critic with a compassionate assertiveness if necessary.

How might that compassionate other/being respond to your critic?

____

____

____

____

e.g. *'Ah now I get why you keep responding to [your name] in this way. It makes sense now I see how this came about in you. This has been hard for you to live your life this way too. But I am here to help [your name] and this* *kind of response is making life incredibly hard for them. So, from now on we are going to be trying some new ways of responding. I will be here to work with you too, so [your name] no longer has to. I understand that you have some fears for [your name] if you were to disappear from her life. I would like to hear about these fears so that I can better help both of you.'*

The response of your compassionate self/compassionate other to the internal self-critic:

____

____

____

____

Reflections on this exercise: What you noticed. What you want to hold onto and remember. What you want to take forward and take action on.

____

____

____

____

It is important that as little attention as possible is focused on working directly with the self-critic as we are aiming to focus instead on growing the compassionate response. (Remember the story of the grandpa, the grandson and the wolves of anger and of self-compassion, when the grandson said, *'Which wolf will win, Grandpa?'* Grandpa replied: *'The wolf that I feed'*.)

The self-critic will begin to fade and disappear naturally over time. But at first the self-critic can be a strong presence which requires us to establish our new position in relation to it, shifting from one of fear to one of assertive compassion.

When we 'feed' our compassionate mind rather than our self-critic, the self-critic will begin to fade and disappear naturally.

But at first the self-critic can be a strong presence which requires us to establish our new position in relation to it, shifting from one of fear to one of assertive compassion.

Reflections and notes: What would you like to take hold of and remember from this section on working with the feelings of unworthiness caused by our inner critic? What would you like to take forward and try? What might be your next steps?

____

____

____

____

Module 51: Letting others (including our baby) take joy and delight in us

As we have seen in this book, a key part in the development of our child's compassionate mind is the building of a particular brain that feels safe, that becomes empathic, can understand the minds of others, can learn and so on. We saw that this isn't just about coming to the aid of our child that is suffering or struggling, but is also about taking joy in them, delighting in them. For them to see in our face that we are glad that they are in this world. These images, sensations, physiological changes, and subsequent brain changes are all part of the development of their compassionate mind.

(We may of course be struggling to experience joy and delight in our child, particularly if we have depression or anxiety. We may also not feel glad they are in the world. It will not be our intention to feel this way, and it makes parenting very hard indeed when we do. If you do feel this way, talk to your GP or health visitor about it. There are now services that can help you.)

Others taking joy in you may not have been your experience as a child, hence the struggle you may be having with feeling loveable, and worthy of care and compassion. However, your baby will be wired to take delight and joy in you, to love your voice and your smell. This is a key part of that 'dance' that parents and babies are wired to engage in. So, if you do feel unlovable, allowing other people, and your baby, to take joy and delight in you is going to be hard, but very important.

How might your compassionate mind help you, step by step, to begin to allow other people, and your baby, to take joy and delight in you, and to display their pleasure that you are in their lives?

(Remember to switch into your compassionate mind first before considering this:

'Body like a mountain, breath like the wind, mind like the blue sky,' warm, kind face and voice. Stepping into the part of you that has great wisdom, strength, courage and a deep commitment to being as helpful and caring as you can.)

____

____

____

____

Exercise: Acting as if you were a being who allows others to take joy and delight in you

With our new brain abilities, we have the capability to be able to pretend we are method acting a person or being (or perhaps a pet or animal) who allows others to take joy in us. Even if we do not believe we can let others take joy in us, we can experiment with acting 'as if' we were such a person.

Imagine you are a method actor who has been studying a person, being or animal who can allow others to take joy in them. You have been studying this person for months; studying how they move, how they sound if they speak, the expression on their face, how they interact with the world and with others around them. Imagine stepping into their body and moving around the room, and interacting with others as you play act this other person or being.

What do you notice? How do you feel? What do you want to take hold of and remember from this?

____

____

____

____

Reflections and notes: What would you like to take hold of and remember from this section on letting others, including our baby, take joy and delight in us? What would you like to take forward and try? What might be your next steps?

____

____

____

____

Module 52: Learning to be playful and joyful

We may have had very little experience of being playful and joyful as a child. But we can see that the ability to play and to experience joy is crucial for our child for many reasons, including building positive memories, a sense of self, of being loveable, enjoyable and capable, and a sense of others as being loving. These experiences grow strong brain systems connected to safeness, steadiness, resilience and confidence, as well as enabling the discovery of new abilities.

Experiences of being playful and joyful are crucial to us as adults too. They occur when we feel safe. For a child this is when somebody else is acting as the 'eyes and ears' for danger, where the parent or other attachment figures are their secure base. When this is in place for us, we can be free too. We can play, be silly, be creative, be joyful. As adults we therefore also need to have a part of ourselves that looks out for us and to begin to trust others to be a secure base for us too.

Think about who and what is your secure base? When do you find it easier to be playful? Who helps you to be more playful?

____

____

____

____

What might help you to be able to be more playful and more joyful? (For example, this may include help with getting treatment for perinatal depression which affects the very areas of our brain which enable us to be joyful and playful.)

We have a gift in the presence of our baby, who is really wanting to be playful too, with us, and with others. But it may be that this is unfamiliar to us and we don't know where to start. (In fact, their wish to play may feel more of a burden than a gift.)

How might your compassionate mind help you with this?

Here are some suggestions:

- There are many internet sites that offer suggestions on playing with our baby. There are some good ideas on websites for grandparents. There are even sites that suggest messy and non-messy, or noisy and quiet versions of activities.
- Books available from libraries and resources available from your health visitor. There may also be local centres that you can attend which will teach play activities or may have a nursery nurse who can help you. There are also programmes that might be run by perinatal and health visiting support services such as 'Watch Me Play' which teach the idea of just watching your baby, delighting in them, and following their lead, and Circle of Security (which looks at how to become the secure base and safe haven for your child).
- Watching others with your baby with curiosity and an intention to learn.
- Gathering ideas from watching others play with their baby.
- Babies love to learn and be part of our world; after all, they are learning the skills to

be able to live in our world, so they often prefer what we are doing to their own toys. Our activities can be a source of play, e.g. helping to cook (having dried rice to pour in and out of containers, a banana to chop with a baby knife when a little older, things to stir, mash, squish), putting washing in and getting it out of washing machine, painting the walls with you (may not be of a great standard!), scribbling on paper as you fill out forms, digging in the garden, weeding and planting with you, playing with sand.

My list of ideas and resources for playing with my baby

____

____

____

____

What for you is being playful as an adult? It could be following dance videos on the internet, singing loudly, painting, cooking, gardening, watching the birds or the clouds, playing a sport, playing video games, playing board games, reading, writing.

____

____

____

____

What ideas do you have from what you enjoy, or used to enjoy, as an adult or child that you might want to try with your child?

____

____

____

____

Method acting: act 'as if' you were a playful person. Imagine you had been studying a joyful, playful person for many months as a method actor: how they move, the expression on their face, how their voice sounds, how they interact with the world and others. Imagine stepping into their body and clothes and then move around the room as them – what does this feel like? What do you notice? What do you want to take hold of and remember from this?

How might your compassionate self or other help you to bring more joy and play into your everyday life?

Reflections and notes: What would you like to take hold of and remember from this section on learning to be playful and joyful? What would you like to take forward and try? What might be your next steps?

Module 53: Using our compassionate mind to help us act assertively (rather than submissively, aggressively or passive-aggressively)

We may have spent a lifetime, until we have our baby, being shaped to get our needs met in certain ways. This can be affected by many factors, including our upbringing, our society's view of how we should behave, and our culture, and can begin shaping us even as young babies. Now that we have our own baby, we might want to respond differently. This can be hard, especially if we have a strong sense of how we *don't* want to be (*'I don't want to shout anymore'*; *'I don't want my baby to think that how I am is the only way of getting what you need or want'*; or, *'I don't want to try and be the nice one who then ends up letting everyone walk all over me. And that might include my baby too actually.'*). We also need a sense of how we *do* want to be. This is where our compassionate guide or mentor comes in. They help us work out what *to* do or how to find out what to do and how we want to be instead.

We may have learned that if we get cross or upset as a child, then this is met with anger, disapproval or a turning away. Whereas if we are 'good' and 'nice' and just put up with it, then people that we rely on to care for us, stay happy, seem to function better, stay with us (mentally and/or physically) and seem more able to look after us. We might learn to become submissive, apologetic. Or to try to keep in our anger or distress by having our critic put us down as soon as anger starts to flicker, or by overeating or using alcohol, for example. We end up harming ourselves in some way or never getting our needs met.

This is a particularly powerful dynamic if we get some sense that for whatever reason our mother cannot cope with us. We learn to delay or inhibit our needs and our protests in order to help her to manage, because we are, at a primal, evolved level, utterly dependent on her for our very lives. So not only do we learn to suppress our needs and our protests, but we might also learn that there is something about our (very normal) way of being that could destroy our mother, leading of course to our annihilation too. We can then carry with us, not just our suppressed anger and needs, but a sense that if we were to become unleashed then we could become destroyers of people we care about and/or depend upon. This may all have begun right from the beginnings of our lives, before we even had words, so we may carry all this at an unconscious level. No wonder we might spend our lives trying to manage our anger.

Our anger might come out in more passive aggressive ways because we fear being fully angry. For example, not telling our partner that something important is happening, knowing they will forget and then have to sort out the consequences.

When we have a baby, we might find that we are using the same strategies, trying to be the 'nice' mum by letting our child always have what they want, never saying 'no', or really diminishing our needs so that we seem to disappear. It can also feel that this is reinforced by the messages that we might be surrounded by about mothers; that when we become a mother we are supposed to become all giving, all loving, completely calm and serene. Inevitably this is not possible, but when our anger does leak out, we still might feel like we have failed, especially if others around us seem to be that way. This can be so difficult because we *do* want to be nice parents and good parents, and our needs necessarily are put to one side because our baby is utterly dependent on us to get their needs met. So how do we find this balance?

This is where our baby can again be our teacher. What do we want for our child as they grow up with regard to getting their needs met and protecting themselves from overwhelming demands of others?

____

____

____

We are likely to want them to be able to do this very difficult dance as best they can; of holding in mind the needs of others, whilst not losing sight of their own needs. To be able to respond not with submission, passive aggressiveness or aggression, but instead with a compassionate assertiveness.

Which are the areas where you would like to be more assertive?

(This might be with your partner, your wider family, at work, in shops, with your child for example.)

____

____

____

____

Pick one to work through as an example:

____

____

What might be getting in the way of you being able to be assertive?

____

____

____

____

These might be fears of how you might respond, for example angry or tearful rather than assertive. Or fears of the person you might become such as somebody who upsets people and ends up alone. It might be about how other people will perceive you or respond to you. Or perhaps you are OK with being able to say what you need to say assertively, rather it is the dealing with a subsequent angry response or argument that you are worried about.

e.g. *'I am worried that if I ask him to help me more, he will get cross and storm off. I hate it when he is like that and I then also end up with even less help.'*

It may be because you are in a relationship where you are truly scared of the consequences of being assertive such as an abusive or coercively controlling relationship. If this is the case, then you are likely to need help and support from organisations, friends and family. The most important thing is that you and your baby are safe.

If you were to imagine yourself behaving in an assertive way, what do you notice?

(This can highlight any fears or blocks or safety issues before trying out any new behaviour for real.)

____

____

____

____

e.g. *'If I imagine standing up straighter, and talking more directly, looking people in the eye, I feel very exposed and I imagine people saying, "What's got into her all of a sudden?" I don't like standing out from the crowd or making a scene and they are not used to me acting this way – they would look at me more.'*

Bring your compassionate self to understanding what might sit behind these fears – how far back did they start? If you were to have voiced your needs and wishes assertively then, what might have happened?

____

____

____

____

e.g. 'When I was little, I was called a show-off if I made a scene, and was really ridiculed. Things were better if I just stayed quiet and unnoticed.'

What did you then need to do, consciously or unconsciously, to make sure these feared consequences of you being assertive didn't happen again? (These are your safety strategies from your formulation.)

___

___

___

___

e.g. 'No wonder then that I tried to just be good and quiet. I would have this voice in my head that would say to me, "Just be quiet, no-one wants to hear from you. If you make a scene, things will be very horrible for you." I suppose I had taken into my own head their very words and manner when I think about it. I realise that voice is still with me now, after all these years.'

Bring your compassionate self or other to your safety strategies and the unintended consequences that may have flowed from them. How would they be towards the fact that you have tried your best over all these years to protect yourself from these feared consequences happening again (and that as humans we are wired to protect ourselves, seek safeness, and avoid threat).

What might they say about your safety strategies and the unintended consequences? How might they understand and validate you?

___

___

___

___

e.g. 'You had to develop these ways of trying to get the best care you could without even realising it, all these years ago. This was no-one's fault really, just everyone doing the best they could with the difficult human mind we all have. But what a hard time you've had as a consequence, having to keep down your liveliness, your playfulness, and energy, as well as keeping all those needs and wants squashed down for all these years. This is not what you would want for your child. And it sounds like it is not what you want for yourself either. I understand how hard and scary it is to do something different though, and that people are used to how you have been. But it is too important to let this go any longer.

I understand that you also want to show your child a different way of being with people. So, we will take this slowly, step by step. And I will be with you, helping, supporting and guiding you every step of the way.'

Just allow yourself, along with your compassionate self or other, to spend a moment to honour your safety strategies. If your safety strategies could be imagined as a part of you that had tried valiantly, with the limited resources they had to hand, to keep you safe. How might you honour them for what they have done? (This is like a retirement ceremony for your safety strategies, as you are looking to leave those safety strategies behind, and find new ways of operating in the world that fit with your current or new life, rather than your old one.)

What might you want to say to this 'safety strategy' part of you?

____

____

____

____

e.g. 'Thank you for all you have done for me. I didn't quite realise just what it was you are doing and why. So often what you did caused me other problems and I would be so angry with you. I hadn't realised that, of course, you come from my threat system, so you only had the tools available in my threat system for you to use, as best you could. All of these years you have worked to make sure my fears didn't happen again. I am going to find new ways of doing this now, which will fit better with the life I now lead, and the new one I want to lead, especially now I have a baby. But I just wanted to honour you and thank you. And now you can retire and rest.'

Allow your compassionate self and compassionate other/image to help you with how this new compassionately assertive response may look and sound:

- It can be helpful to start with a clear statement of what it is you need (this can help to really clarify it in your own mind too, e.g. When . . . , I feel . . . , I need . . . , I would like . . . – hold both yourself and the other person with your wise, caring, courageous, compassionate mind).

- Then express why this is important to you, and what you would like from the other person.
- Just holding in mind if you were asking yourself this in this manner, how it feels to you. In other words, avoiding blame, shame, submissive or passive-aggressive tones, anything that switches the threat system rather than the compassion system on. Perhaps inviting them, or asking if they would be willing . . . Any language and tone that understands and has a sense of connection for both of you, the wanting to resolve it together, and for each other, the understanding of the struggles and background that have led to the both of you arriving here in this moment, in this manner.

An example of a compassionately assertive response that you may try out:

e.g. 'When you come home from work, both of us are exhausted and we are trying to do such a lot, just the two of us, now we have our baby. I know I feel so exhausted that I get cross with you. Doing all the evening tasks feels like a mountain that I cannot carry on climbing. Really it is too much for us both. I have realised I need some help with all this. I think we probably both do. Can we think together about what would make the evenings easier for both of us? Then perhaps we can find time to just sit and watch something together before I go to bed as I really miss having that time with you. In fact, I miss you!'

Actually trying this out can be challenging; after all, there have been very good reasons why you've found it hard to be assertive for all these years. So, like anything that is challenging and new, your compassionate self and compassionate other can help you with this, just as you would help your child learn something new and challenging. These are some ideas that your compassionate self and compassionate other might suggest:

- Write a compassionate letter to yourself from your compassionate self or other to help clarify and understand what is happening now for you, why it is important for you to try to do things differently, understand why it has been so hard to do this in the past, and how they can help you with this now. (See compassionate letter writing.)

What might your compassionate self or other write? (Just jot down some rough notes of what it might include here. You can write this in full too if you wish.)

____

____

Imagine role playing this assertive version of yourself – like a method actor – imagining stepping into the body of your assertive self, the clothes you would wear, how you would hold your body, how your body would move, your feeling of steadiness and stability, your slow, calm breath, the expression on your face and the sound of your voice, your warmth, kindness, helpfulness, commitment to caring, courage, wisdom and strength. Notice what you 'bump into' during your day as you imagine acting as this person. This can help identify any areas that might derail you, that your compassionate self or compassionate other can then help you with.

What is this like as you imagine role-playing this assertive version of yourself? What do you notice? What would you like to take hold of and remember from this? What might you like to take forward and begin working with?

Practice: Compassionate body swap

- Sit (or stand) in your 'dignified' posture, feet hip width apart, flat on the ground, back and head upright. Bring your shoulders up to your ears, then drop them back and down, feeling the openness in your chest. Bring your warm, kind face and voice to your breath, perhaps in your mind saying, 'Hello breath!' Allowing your in breath and your out breath to begin to slow down. Let your breathing find its own soothing rhythm. As it does, you might notice your body feeling a little sturdier, a little steadier and more stable.
- Move into that part of you that has great strength and courage, that is wise, that is committed to being as helpful and compassionate as it can.
- Now bring to mind a scenario where you have struggled to be assertive. Notice who is there, what is happening, how you feel.

The scenario I am struggling with is:

___

___

___

___

- Imagine stepping outside of the scenario and watching it from above, from your wise, kind, strong, courageous, compassionate mind.

What strikes you when viewing this from this new perspective?

___

___

___

___

- Now imagine that a compassionate figure arrives – perhaps your compassionate other, a wise, strong, perhaps ancient compassionate being who has been dealing with difficult things for years, perhaps hundreds of years. They say to you, 'Can I help you with this?' You watch how they deal with this situation. How they move, how they speak, how they interact with the other person.

What do you notice?

____

____

____

____

- Then they invite you to swap clothes and body with them. You step into their strength, their courage, their wisdom and compassion. You notice how you walk, how you talk, how your body feels, how you interact with those around you. Notice then how you deal with this situation as this compassionate being.

What do you notice?

____

____

____

____

End of practice.

Your reflections and notes on this practice. What would you like to hold onto and remember from this practice?

____

____

____

____

- Write what you want to do and say on a postcard and just carry it round with you in your pocket for a few days. This helps us to imagine how it might feel to begin thinking and behaving in this way.
- Recruit other people to help you. Perhaps tell a friend or colleague at work, or family member, that you are going to try this out. Role play it with them, or ask their advice and their help.
- Try this on small things, or when it is easier – perhaps at first imagining what you'd like to say rather than actually saying it, like quietly trying on some clothes that you wouldn't normally wear in the changing room while no-one is looking.
- It may be enough to just not say or do what you would normally say or do, like refusing to keep doing your part of the 'dance' that has happened between you and a parent for most of your life. You might notice your heart pounding because both of you know at some level what you should be saying or doing right now. These might just be minute ways of holding your body differently or pausing slightly longer than you would normally before saying what you are expected to say. These are tiny rebellions, but rebellions all the same, and are an important stage in making changes. Both parties can discover that life doesn't fall apart when the dance happens a little differently.
- Use your compassionate self or other to help the other person with this change too. Your family, your partner, your friends, your work colleagues, even your child, have learned particular patterns and ways of being with you. You are changing the dance, even if it is by an almost imperceptible amount so the other person will be slightly out of step too. You might want to explicitly tell people that you are trying out something different.

How might you help the people around you to understand and adapt as you try out your new compassionate assertiveness?

____

____

____

____

e.g. 'I know, I don't usually say things like that, do I! It's all a bit strange for me, and probably for you too, but I am giving it a go. I really think this might be a better way of being now, but I am going to be a bit clunky and clumsy at the beginning. I am just learning this and might need a bit of help.'

They might need time to adjust their dance too and catch up with you, but in the meantime, it might be a bit bumpy and strange for all involved so lean on your compassionate self or other to help you through this bit.

- We cannot of course control how others are going to respond, even if we do our very best. You are learning something new and tricky and will almost certainly trip up and have it all come out wrong at first. So, you also need your compassionate self and other helping you with any of the tricky outcomes – e.g. getting an angry and defensive response from people, being noticed when you are used to hiding away, having to try out a new way of being whilst wondering whether over time people won't like this version of you.
- Write out below how your compassionate self or compassionate other might help you with any difficulties or setbacks. Imagine you are helping your child to get through setbacks – what might you say? Knowing how we will get through even when things go very wrong, is a key part of us feeling able to give it a go in the first place – so this 'What if the setbacks or difficulties do happen' plan is very important. Knowing we will get through even the most challenging of setbacks means we can keep picking ourselves back up and carrying on rather than giving up and going back to our old ways.

What will help me if this worst-case scenario happens:

____

____

____

____

This is why I am doing this – this is what is important to me (this is like putting a flag on a distant mountain to keep reminding yourself of where you are heading to and why):

____

____

____

____

Reflections and notes: What would you like to take hold of and remember from this section on learning how to be compassionately assertive? What would you like to take forward and try? What might be your next steps?

____

____

____

____

SECTION 8:

Using our compassionate mind to help us with difficult feelings

Module 54: Anger

Uncharacteristic feelings of anger and rage during pregnancy or postnatally can be symptoms of rapid hormonal changes, particularly, but not exclusively, in women who have suffered from strong mood changes connected to their menstrual period. Anger can be a symptom of other factors such as depression and post-traumatic stress disorder. It is also commonly linked to poor maternal sleep, helplessness around sleep, and to factors such as a loss of personal autonomy, compromised needs such a loss of adequate nutrition or of what ordinarily keeps us in balance, and of loss of support from within the family and/or from the wider community. Bearing in mind too that we are also wired to require support to look after our baby, feeling judged or criticised, or feeling we may lose support, for example, can trigger levels of anger that we previously hadn't experienced prior to becoming pregnant or having our baby. Our hormones, particularly those connected to breastfeeding, can also enhance feelings of protectiveness towards our baby which may also trigger levels of anger towards others that we are not used to. These are just a few examples of what may lead to high levels of anger in the perinatal period.

When we are surrounded by images of the archetypal mother as calm, doting, forever loving and selflessly giving, it can be extremely difficult when we experience rage, hostility or dislike in relation to our baby. However, these feelings are more common than we might imagine. Because these are often not talked about, this can make us feel scared and ashamed when we feel them. If we could share them with others, we are likely to find understanding, connection and help if we need it. It is as if these 'dark' feelings deepen when kept in the dark. When we bring them into the open, into the light if you like, then they often lose their power or disappear completely. But this can be so scary to do. Especially if we fear being shamed or looked down on, or abandoned by people, especially the people we need. We might fear that we will be judged as unfit to care for our baby. And of course, as we know, this is our great evolved fear as humans; that for most of our evolved lives as humans, being cast out of the group would have almost certainly meant we would have died. And for women in the perinatal period this evolved wiring to need others seems to be turned up even further. So, it is no wonder we might have such fear in telling people how we are feeling towards our baby or others. But telling people (including ourselves) is the way towards help, relief and resolution.

Sometimes, particularly if we are experiencing severe depression, bipolar disorder, postpartum psychosis, extreme hormonal changes, or feel trapped by our baby with no way out, we may have the urge to actually harm our baby, or ourselves, or both the baby and ourselves. If you feel this way, it is important to ensure that your baby is somewhere safe and then seek help immediately by calling the emergency services (999 in the UK). You may wish to contact somebody you trust instead, such as a friend or family member, your midwife, health visitor or GP, but make sure they understand any imminent risk to you or your baby (or both of you). These feelings after having a baby are understood by services and we are well-provisioned in the UK (and may be too in other countries) with Mother and Baby units where you can go with your baby for help with just these kinds of experiences. Your baby can be cared for by the staff if necessary while you receive care and treatment. The vast majority of mothers develop a good bond with their baby and these feelings disappear, despite most mothers believing that their feelings will never change and seeing no way out. Very occasionally, the parents might decide that fostering or adoption of the baby might be the best outcome. This can be done sensitively and carefully if this does indeed seem to be the best way forward. Whatever happens, there is good help available, and these feelings will pass.

We are going to look at how to manage anger using the compassionate mind approach, but as part of this we can bring the wide-angle lens and curious part of our compassionate mind to look at factors triggering our anger that we might not have previously considered.

As we looked at earlier, being angry can be a common fear in women. In particular societies and cultures, girls are valued for being quiet, nice, submissive and non-confrontational, and shamed or disapproved of for being angry or standing up for themselves. Sometimes it can even be dangerous for women or girls to express their anger or be assertive. This can be exacerbated when we become mothers by images and cultural views of how a good mother should be: patient, calm, all giving, non-demanding and selfless.

It is common to hear women say, 'I don't do anger' or 'I don't like anger'. However, we, like our babies, are born with the ability to be angry, so what happens to that anger as we grow up?

If we could remove that emotion from our baby, would we? What would it be like for our baby to grow up and go through life without the ability to be angry?

____

____

____

____

What are some of your fears in being angry?

A fear that we might have in addressing this is that our pent-up anger will be unleashed, and we will end up destroying relationships or harming people. This can become an even greater fear when we have a baby and feel and see the difference between our baby's vulnerability, smallness and trust in us, and our size, strength and potential to harm our baby. Mothers can end up working even harder to suppress their anger. But with tiredness, overwhelm, anxiety and the relentless demands of parenthood, inevitably frustration and anger leak out as mothers are only human too.

Anger may be overlaying an even deeper feeling – one of grief. Sometimes when we are working with our fears, it can be like pulling on a fishing line – we think we have got to the thing that is weighty and pulling us, for example the anger, but there is still more. Often, beyond our anger, we find our grief.

Our main threat emotions are anxiety, anger, and sadness or grief. But from our work on the many parts of us (see 'multiple selves' section) we can see that we often have one emotion that we are comfortable with, often the one that it was safest to feel as a child, and another emotion that is the hardest or scariest for us to feel – perhaps one we were shamed for or that a parent couldn't cope with, so withdrew their love and care of us when we exhibited it. Grief can be the emotion that is most deeply buried – perhaps grief for the love and care that we never got, or a parent that wasn't or couldn't be there for us, or the childhood that we never had. This is dealt with in more detail below, but it is mentioned here because sometimes our intuitive wisdom stops us from dealing with one thing such as anger, because it knows, even subconsciously, that there is a deeper, much harder to deal with emotion that would be pulled up once we face the first. If this is the case, then we might need to visit the section on fear of grief (below) first.

Anger may be overlaying an even deeper feeling – one of grief.

If you could overcome your fear of anger, how might it help you?

How might things be different for you if you could have your anger as part of your life?

Why might this be important to you?

From our formulation, we can identify the safety strategies that we have learned to use to keep the anger in, such as attacking ourselves with our self-critic, overeating, cleaning the house obsessively, and we can end up doubling-down on our safety strategies when our baby comes along.

So how do we behave differently when we feel angry after perhaps even a lifetime of trying not to be angry? Again, our baby can be our guide.

When your baby gets angry, what are some unhelpful responses towards them? How might you make them even crosser?

Think about the last time your baby expressed frustration, annoyance or anger.

If that frustrated or angry part of your baby could appear in front of you, what might it say it was bothered about?

What might happen if you ignored it or tried to distract it?

What might happen if you criticised it or got cross with it?

____

____

____

____

What does it really need to help settle it?

____

____

____

____

What does your baby really need instead? What might be some helpful responses? What would help to settle them?

____

____

____

____

Now step into your compassionate self (sitting or standing with your feet hip width apart, steady and stable, shoulders back and down, slowing down your in and out breath, breathing deeply and smoothly in and out from the base of your lungs, bringing a warm, kind face and warm, kind voice, along with your wise mind, your commitment to being as helpful as you can, your strength and your courage).

Does anything else come to mind about what your baby really needs when they are angry? Any other helpful responses? Anything else that might help here?

____

____

____

____

Now imagine your compassionate image arriving. How might they be with both you and your baby? How might they help you both?

____

____

____

____

When you get angry, what are some unhelpful responses towards you?

____

____

____

____

Think about the last time you felt angry.

If that angry part could be seated in front of you, what would it say it was bothered about?

____

____

____

____

What would happen if you tried to ignore or criticise that angry part?

____

____

____

____

What does that angry part really need? What would really help it to settle down?

____

____

____

____

What do you really need instead? What might be some helpful responses? What would help to settle you?

____

____

____

____

We can see here that the emotional patterns or 'parts' within ourselves and within our baby are not very different. What we want, and what our baby wants, is to be turned to, listened to in a steady, containing manner rather than with anxiety or crossness, validated ('Gosh, this has really upset you, hasn't it? I can get why you are so cross about this'), and then for an attempt to be made to help us. This help might be just sitting there with our own or our baby's discomfort so they, and we, don't have to bear it alone, even if we can't actually take the discomfort away.

Imagine that the angry part of you was seated in another chair, and you could talk to it or interview it with genuine curiosity and warmth – you really want to understand it and come to know it.

What would it tell you about what is going on for it at the moment?

____

____

____

____

What has it been struggling with lately? What is making it feel more angry than usual?

____

____

____

____

When does it feel a little more settled?

____

____

____

____

What is its fear for you if it were to disappear just when you needed it?

What other part steps in to intercept this angry part and stop it letting you know how it feels? (Perhaps the self-critic, or a shaming part, a flippant or jokey part, a cut-off or squashing down part, or a tearful or anxious part.)

How do you feel towards it when you hear all of this? What might you want to say to it? What might be your heartfelt wish for it?

How might you help it from now on in?

Imagine you are a method actor who has been studying a person who is compassionate to their own anger, for many months: how they move, how they sound if they speak, the expression on their face, how they interact with others. Now imagine stepping into this character and method acting 'as if' you are them. Notice how your body changes, your posture, how you move, how you sound, the expressions on your face, how you are in the world, how you interact with others.

How do you feel? What do you notice?

You might have noticed some of these aspects that were important for both your baby and you:

1. The importance of feeling steady and grounded – anger can make us scared and want to run away or to become bigger, louder and scarier ourselves, so we need to find steadiness, strength and inner calmness and courage in our body first.
2. We are facing towards the angry person with a clear intention of trying to find a way through in as helpful a way as possible rather than to attack, criticise, destroy or humiliate.
3. We use our empathy to understand what the other person needs – we may want to cuddle them or shush them, or stop them being upset and angry, but they may want to keep a bit of physical space and to be allowed to express just what it is they are angry about.
4. Validation is key, even for a pre-verbal baby. So, express that you can see their anger and you understand it (or are trying to understand it as best you can). That it isn't

being minimised, shamed or dismissed; e.g. to your baby, *'You really wanted to rip your sister's painting, didn't you? And you are very mad that I pulled it out of your hands so sharply. It made you jump, and made you very cross, didn't it? I am sorry I pulled it from you so quickly, but I really didn't want you to rip it.'* Your voice tone and facial expression will be conveying so much, even to your baby when they may not understand your words.

5. Taking action from a place of compassion: Validation is so powerful that sometimes that can be enough as we feel met in our distress, understood and safe. Sometimes however action is needed. So, with our baby we might pick them up once they are calm enough, cuddle them, perhaps get them involved in something else. We might also take note of what we can do to avoid or head off this situation in the future.

   If *we* are angry, then validating us might be enough, but perhaps we also need the person to demonstrate that they are sorry, that they have taken what we had to say seriously and are making changes for the future, for example.

6. We might also want to help our baby to deal with the situation differently in the future, and we might need similar help ourselves. This is where we can become a compassionate teacher or guide to our child and why we might need a compassionate guide ourselves. Our compassionate guide is important in letting us know if we are going a bit too far, or that we might need to go and apologise and make things right with that person. We are taking our responsibility for dealing with our anger seriously, particularly now we have a baby, and we need to know that we have a skilful presence to guide us.

   Knowing we have our compassionate self or guide brings a safeness that we don't have without it. We know it truly has our best interests at heart. It won't be nice to us to be liked, like a friend who won't tell the truth about whether we've upset someone when we've asked for their advice, for fear we will get annoyed with them. Instead, it will be like the true friend who genuinely wants the best for us even if something is hard for them to say, and for us to take. This friend ends up being the one we can lean on and trust, which is what gives us that safeness. This is what our compassionate self or guide brings to us in terms of behaviour; we know it will help to be a trustworthy and honest guide to us. This enables us to tentatively pick up anger and start to allow it into our lives in a helpful way.

Reflections and notes: What would you like to take hold of and remember from this section on bringing our compassionate mind to our struggles with anger? What would you like to take forward and try? What might be your next steps?

____

____

____

____

Module 55: Grief and sadness

As we saw above in the working with anger section, grief can be a deep and painful emotion that lies underneath our anger and our anxiety. Grief is the loss of something that is important to us. It pulls us to try to find what we have lost and gives us a feeling of distress if we cannot get it back.

When has your child experienced grief? What might cause their grief?

____

____

____

____

e.g. 'He definitely experienced grief when we left his favourite teddy behind on the bus. That was all he could focus on for ages.' 'She was upset for a long time when her big brother started school. She missed him so much.' 'He seemed so sad when we couldn't go to the playgroup anymore. He cried and cried if we went on the same route that we used to take to get there.'

What does your child need when they are experiencing grief? What might help them?

____

____

____

____

e.g. 'All I could do was to keep cuddling him and consoling him.' 'I tried to do nice things with her and tried to buy her a new toy. It would work for a while but then the grief came back. I just had to cuddle and be there for her. After a long while it got less until she hardly talks about it now. I just had to find a way of hanging on in there. It was quite hard work at times to be honest.'

If you imagine allowing your grief to come to the surface, what would that be like?

____

____

____

____

Does it feel OK or are there any fears, blocks or resistances to letting your grief come to the surface?

____

____

____

____

e.g. 'I fear that if I start crying, there is so much inside of me that I will never stop. Or perhaps it would send me mad.' 'I fear that people would be dismayed and not want to be around me.' 'I worry that that is not how they see me – I am the one that consoles everybody else. I will lose my role and my sense of who I am, and they will not like this version of me either.' 'No-one will come. I will be left alone in all this grief.'

How might your compassionate self or other validate your fears, blocks or resistances to your grief? What might they say or do?

____

____

____

____

e.g. 'How hard is that, to carry that immense sadness and grief around with you for so much of your life. And not just the grief, but the fear of what might happen if you let it out.'

How might your compassionate self or other help you to understand how these fears, blocks or resistances have developed in relation to grief? What might they say or do?

____

____

____

____

e.g. 'It is no wonder you fear that you will be left alone in your grief – because that is what happened. Your father really struggled with tears, and he was grieving himself for when his mother, your dear grandmother, died. He just didn't know what to do with you so he would give you sweets, put the TV on and go and busy himself elsewhere. He was very kind to you, but he was struggling and lost and tried to deal with you the best way he could, but ended up leaving you alone with your sadness and grief.'

What would have helped you instead? What did you need that would have meant that it was OK to be grieving and sad?

____

____

____

____

e.g. 'I wish that somebody could have helped my dad and showed him that all he needed to do was to cuddle me and be with me. I know that I would have needed a lot of that, and Dad was on his own, and very sad himself, but it would have helped me so much, and eventually I wouldn't have needed so many cuddles. Then I would know that the grief comes and goes, even from moment to moment, that it is horrible but bearable, that it gets better over time, and isn't anything to be feared, just a consequence of loving and caring for people. Then I would be more prepared to let myself love people, including my baby, knowing that I could bear the grief if I was to lose them.'

How might your compassionate self or other help you to begin to be with your grief and sadness?

___

___

___

___

For example:

- Write you a compassionate letter.
- Help you to have time when you can just cry.
- Remind you that you know very well how to put away your grief and sadness, after all you have spent a lifetime honing these skills, so you can use these familiar skills to let the grief out bit by bit whenever you have the space, and then put it away again, allowing the 'pool' of grief to get smaller and smaller over time. You don't need to somehow find space that is big enough to let out all of your grief in one go.
- Help you to discover that grief and sadness are not endless even though if feels that way – given all the time and space in the world in the end we run out of tears, even becoming bored of our own tears. We are wired to habituate (get used to) anything that is no longer new and different. That is not to say the tears won't come again, but we can learn that grief and sadness come and go, like clouds passing over, and we can bear it each time.
- Help you to remember that what your child wants the most is for you to be there for them, even if they are grieving for something or someone else that you can't bring back. So, like our child, we still need to turn up for ourselves, in a compassionate rather than frustrated, or panicky way, and just be with ourselves again and again.
- Help you to begin to ask others you care about to be with you and to hear about your grief, and to witness it too. They might need help in knowing that there is nothing complicated that they need to do – just listen and be there for you.
- Help you to create in your own life what you lost, e.g. being loved and cared for, being

delighted in, being free, playful, joyful, silly. We might give it to ourselves from our compassionate mind or compassionate other or seek out others who can give us this or help us experience this.

- Help you to seek out a fuller story of your childhood or of what you have missed – perhaps talking to others about their memories, gathering photos.

Imagine if your grief or sadness were to sit on another chair and you can talk to it or interview it with a warm, compassionate curiosity – you really want to get to know it a little better.

What might it tell you?

Perhaps it might talk about when the grief or sadness felt easier, and when it began to feel more difficult.

Perhaps it would tell you what it fears for you if it could no longer be around. It might have noticed that when it tries to come up in you then another part of you steps in and blocks it or squashes it down – perhaps the self-critic, or anger, anxiety, shame or a shutting down part.

You might want to find out what it really needs. What really helps it.

You might notice how you feel towards it.

Perhaps you notice your heartfelt wish for it.

There may be something you want to tell it, or a particular way you want to be with it.

Perhaps you notice how you would like to begin to help it going forward from here.

Imagine you are a method actor who, for many months, has been studying a person who can respond to their own grief and sadness with compassion: how they move, how they sound if they speak, the expression on their face, how they interact with others. Now imagine stepping into this character and method acting 'as if' you are them. Notice how your body changes, your posture, how you move, how you sound, the expressions on your face, how you are in the world, how you interact with others.

How do you feel? What do you notice?

Your reflections on this section – what would you like to hold onto from this?

Grief in parenthood to non-death losses

Parenthood is such a time of rapid change. And with change comes both gains, but also losses. We quickly lose the tininess of our baby and have to put away their first vests. We lose their gummy smile when they get their first tooth. We lose their newborn hair when it rubs off on their mattress, and then their longer hair when they have their first haircut. We lose their closeness when they feed themselves, and lose our milk when we finish breastfeeding. We lose the cuddles when they don't want to cuddle us much anymore. We lose their toddling walk and the funny way they say words. How do we bear this endless change with so many losses?

We may lose aspects of ourselves, perhaps temporarily or permanently. For example, our freedom to just leave the house when we wish, friends who don't have children, hobbies or activities that keep us feeling regulated, for example running or reading. We may lose our familiar body or the functioning of our bladder. We may lose ideas or beliefs that become shattered, such as a belief that we are fertile or that we are having a boy when in fact it's a girl (or vice versa), that there is a 'just world' and that our life of being a good person and doing everything as right as we can, will mean that we will have a baby. That the baby we had would not be the one we have had.

This is part of the significance of the cherry blossom in Japan – awaiting its beauty for so long, but when it arrives experiencing the bitter-sweet feeling of knowing it will soon be gone again. It is a symbol of how we might learn to hold the impermanence of life with lightness and ease, with a looseness rather than gripping hold tightly of the good and pushing away the bad. This is known as 'equanimity' – trying to allow both the good and the bad equally as if they were resting on our hand like butterflies, neither holding them tightly nor forcing them away. It is a sense of allowing with warmth, wisdom, understanding and curiosity. Our baby as they grow inadvertently becomes our teacher about impermanence and change and how we can learn best to be with it.

Practising mindfulness helps us with the sense of just allowing what is there and letting it come and go whilst helping ourselves to sustain this compassionate presence to our grief even if it feels like it is going on for a very long time. (See the section on mindfulness.)

Your notes and reflections on grief in parenthood to non-death losses:

Grief in parenthood to death losses

The loss of a baby during or after pregnancy is usually devastating. There is the loss of so much, including an entire future which we assumed would reach out beyond our own lives; the experiences we would share with them, the toys we have saved for them from our childhood, the wedding we may have hoped to organise with them, the grandchildren we may have imagined, the helping them with their first home. There may be a shattering of the sense of the robustness of life; that once born we are here until old age, and with that may be a great anxiety about how to keep everybody safe and alive. There is also a deeply physical loss, particularly for the mother who, through the process of pregnancy, has undergone huge physiological changes in both her body, but also in her brain. She has been shaped by the process of pregnancy to have a brain ready to experience delight and communication, breasts ready to feed, hormones ready for physical closeness, arms ready to hold, brain wanting to connect. Her brain remains changed and she also contains foetal cells from her baby in her blood, heart, lungs, bones and other organs, which remain for years and maybe forever. These foetal cells are affecting her in numerous ways which are only just being discovered.

Cells from the mother are also passed into the foetus so the mother and baby remain entwined even after baby loss. The cells from the foetus can pass into subsequent brothers and sisters. It is no wonder many mothers feel baby loss as such a visceral and bodily experience.

Parents may deal with their shared loss quite differently and require different things of each other, and from others.

Grandparents may be struggling with the loss of their grandchild and the stories and fantasies that came with that.

A twin may struggle with the loss of their sibling and the attachment relationship that began in the womb. They also experience the transfer of cells between each other so literally carry the DNA of the other within them.

Older siblings may struggle with their loss of a new baby and of becoming the eldest or a member of a larger family.

We may have to be parenting a child when we have lost a baby, or parenting a single twin when we know there should be two, or leaving hospital with no baby at all.

We may then have a baby whilst still grieving the loss of a previous baby, trying to disentangle feelings of grief, anger or disappointment that this new baby isn't the previous one. This may be a lifelong wound that gets repeatedly pulled at each time we see our child reaching milestones that the baby that died will never reach. We may have to bear a much deeper sense of 'sibling rivalry' in this child, or in all of our children, that they exist when, or perhaps because, another baby has died (*'If they had lived then you wouldn't have had me'*).

Even though a baby or a significant relationship is no longer part of our lives, it doesn't mean the relationship ends. We can still feel a physical attachment and have a relationship with the memory of them as well as with the imagined life. This is why people can experience chronic sorrow to losses. The difficulty can be when people feel *'you should be over it by now'* or *'But now you have a baby who is alive and actually here so you should be grateful and focus on them'*. When what people say doesn't resonate with our own experience we can feel very alone.

And the problem can be also that if we don't really understand why we are finding this so hard and prolonged ourselves, then we end up leaving ourselves alone too.

If grief is about loss of connection and relationships, then the healing from grief is about connections rather than disconnection. We might need to find people who do understand us, perhaps through support groups or counselling. We might need to find a way of being very clear with our loved ones about what helps us and how they might help.

We might also need to practise coming to, and connecting with, ourselves. As this is a deeply physical loss, then practices that focus on physical connection with ourselves can be particularly helpful. Our way of being with ourselves is about finding a way of sustaining our compassionate presence to ourselves over what might be a long time. We live in a society where we have become able to cure many things and can get our needs met quickly. However, when there is no cure, then we come back to the concept of care instead; for most of our evolved lives as humans we would only be able to give care rather than cure, and we would be more familiar with how we bear prolonged pain when there is no way to alleviate it.

A compassionate caring presence is very powerful and can alleviate a great deal of suffering even in the absence of curing the suffering. Just think of when our child hurts themselves.

We cannot mend the wound or stop it hurting, but our manner of being with our child helps them immeasurably in being able to bear the pain. When we practise compassion, we are able to sustain a motivation to sit with even prolonged and intense suffering, and the recipient (who may be ourselves) is better able to bear their pain and to experience less pain and suffering. It really is quite remarkable.

Practice: Bringing a sustaining and compassionate presence to our grief and sorrow

- Take a seat (as with all practices, we can adapt this to standing up or walking around, as we need to access our compassionate mind when we are on the go 'in real life' particularly as grief can come upon us sometimes when we least expect it).
- Place your feet hip width apart and feel them making contact with the ground. (This groundedness is important as grief can take us off into our memories of the past and fantasies of the future. We need to have a sense of our secure base so we can go off but come back again or reach out from this place of steadiness and safeness.)
- Sit with your 'dignified' posture ('body like a mountain or mighty oak tree'). Bring your shoulders up to your ears, then drop them down and back, feeling the spaciousness and openness in your body. (Our posture of strength, steadiness, and stability helps us to tap into our courage to be able to go towards and stay with our difficult feelings. It is also what will allow us to sustain this compassionate presence even when other people, or other parts of ourselves – such as our anxious part, or our critic – have given up and left us alone.)
- Bring your warm, kind face and warm, kind voice to this practice. Perhaps imagine greeting yourself as if you are really pleased to see yourself, even when you are upset. You might imagine saying 'Hello' and your name. (We are switching on our system of affiliation, connection and safeness which is so important when we have experienced loss, including the additional loss that occurs when people don't know how to be with us. We are now showing up for ourselves, and our own system will respond as it would to a 'real' person showing up in this way.)

- Bring your warm, kind face and voice to your breath. Perhaps greeting it, 'Hello breath'. You might have a sense of your gratitude and awe that despite these major changes, losses, the rollercoaster of life, our breath is always with us, night and day, sustaining us quietly in the background. Our breath can be a wonderful anchor and key part of our sense of our secure base – our 'port in the storm', a place to come back to of quiet predictability, rhythm and sustenance.
- Allow your in breath to lengthen, breathing in smoothly and deeply to the base of your lungs, notice the pause and then allow your out breath to slowly flow out all the way from the base of your lungs, out into the air. Breathing in and out gently, slowly and smoothly, allowing your breathing to find its own soothing rhythm. As it does, you might notice a sense of your body slowing down and settling. A sense of your body feeling steadier and more stable.
- Move into that part of you that has a deep wish to be as helpful and as caring to yourself as you can. Become aware of your wisdom, developed over years of different experiences, from all of the people you have met, been taught by, or whose words you have read in books or heard in films or on TV, for example. You might notice your awareness that we did not choose these human minds, brains and bodies. We did not choose that we have evolved to be highly social, to be driven to connect, to have an ability to imagine, so that we can make strong bonds and then also create an imagined future together. We never chose any of this. We never chose to have the emotions of grief, yearning, sadness and sorrow, nor the ability to have a critic which can criticise ourselves for it. Our wise mind understands this, that these are not our fault.
- Allow in your strength and courage; these qualities that have meant that you can face difficult things and keep getting back up even when you get knocked down by life repeatedly.
- Bring your warm, kind compassionate mind to take in how you are feeling, noticing where in your body you feel your grief and your sorrow. Bring your warm, caring, mindful attention to this place, perhaps imagining it as a colour, mist or physical sensation of warmth that soaks into this sore place, perhaps like the feeling of placing a hot water bottle on sore muscles.

- Try bringing your hand and placing it over or on this place that feels the pain. Notice the feel of this. Notice the rhythm of the movement of your hand as you breathe.
- Become aware of the sensation of the grief. If you could draw round it, where are the outer edges of where you feel it in your body? What colour or colours would it be if it had colours? What sound might it make if it had a sound? How do these sensations, sounds and colours move and change? Is there a sense of them staying static or do they flow around, wax and wane, come and go, get more intense and less intense?
- Your mindful attention allows these sensations to come and go, to be just as they need to be. There is no expectation that they should be any different.
- The quality of your attention to this pain is like that of a gentle hand that is just resting on, stroking, soothing an area of hurt in your child. You might hear soothing words come to your mind. Just notice these words and take them in.
- If the feelings begin to give you the sense that they will overwhelm you, come back to the secure base of your breath, to the strength and steadiness of your compassionate mind, to your courage, and your wisdom, your knowledge that no matter how large and overwhelming these emotions seem, they will run their course and will pass through us and away ('This too shall pass') . While they are with us, we can bear them. Connect back into your compassionate mind, and imagine your grief seated in front of you. Then sit with it once again.
- Our compassionate mind enables us to be both steady and flexible; able to be grounded, but also to move with the changing flow of our emotions.
- Stay with your grief in this manner as long as you wish.
- When it's time to finish the practice, imagine tucking the grief part of you into your pocket or bringing it alongside you, like a teacher who sits an upset child next to them at their desk and asks them to sharpen the pencils for them. So that you can carry on with your day but still give that grieving part a sense of your steady, compassionate presence – a feeling that you have 'got it' even when you are doing other things. A sense of journeying alongside, letting the grief unfold and come and go in the company of a compassionate mind.

- When you are ready, bring your attention to the sounds in the room, just allowing them to come in through your ears. Bring your attention to the feel of your feet in contact with this ground, perhaps moving them. Become aware of the feel of your hands in your lap, perhaps flexing them. Notice the feel of the chair underneath you, supporting you. When you are ready, gently open your eyes. Stretch if you need to. Take your compassionate mind and body with you as best you can as you move into the next part of your day.

End of practice.

Your notes and reflections on this practice:

Adaptation of previous practices for grief:

Compassionate place for grief: (see compassionate place practice)

- Allow the compassionate place to hold you and take care of you, letting you be just as you need to be. You might bring in your grief, or wish to be here free of grief, or to experience the ebb and flow of it in this place of ease, freedom and support.
- You might come with the baby that died, and have this place allow you to be just as you need to be with your baby.
- You might come with all of your family, including the baby that died.
- Or you may wish just to be alone, or to be with your partner or just with your pet. This is your place. It is here just for you, however you need it to be.

Compassionate letter ideas for grief: (see section on compassionate letter writing)

- Write a letter from your compassionate self or compassionate other to you about your loss and your grief.
- Write a compassionate letter to your baby that died, or to yourself and the baby that died.
- Write a compassionate letter to your partner or your parents about their loss and grief.
- Write a compassionate letter to the child or children that are living.

(Do whatever is helpful to you with the letters once written.)

Compassionate connection between couples after baby loss

The feeling of aloneness between partners who have shared a baby loss is exceedingly common and can be hard to overcome. There can be other emotions and beliefs that can further widen any divide. There can be envy, for example the partner who did not carry the baby envying the deep connection their partner still seems to have with the baby who died, or envy from the mother that her partner can seem to disconnect so easily and go about their life again so quickly after the loss of their baby. There can be secret or overt blame that the mother somehow caused the loss of the baby in her body, or that the actions of the other partner caused the baby loss.

Couples counselling can be very helpful to have a space where both can talk openly in a neutral environment about what they are carrying. However we do it, ultimately the aim is to come to face each other again, and reconnect as a supportive pair who are back on the same path through life (although, like a real walk, we walk together but never exactly in each other's footsteps).

As we now know, the neurophysiological effect of compassionate mind practices shifts our brain and our body into a state which enables us to do many different things compared to when we are in our threat mind, including being able to see the bigger picture and focusing us on connections between us and our partner rather than on divisions and differences between us. It also helps us to integrate new information so enabling us to accept and adapt to this new place we both have moved to in our lives.

What follows is a very powerful practice which can be challenging to do but can have a long-term impact. The aim is to do this with your partner, sitting facing each other either with both of you having your eyes shut, or both looking into each other's eyes, or alternating between one opening their eyes and the other opening their eyes. You may want to make physical contact such as sit knee to knee, next to each other or holding hands for example. It is a very intense practice but can be very moving and profoundly impactful on couples. However, even practising this on our own can have a deep impact on our relationship with our partner.

Practice: Fostering compassionate connection between a couple following baby loss

- Sit with your eyes closed or looking at your partner, or perhaps looking at a photo or object that represents your partner. Sit upright in your 'dignified' posture, with your feet hip width apart, shoulders dropped back and down, head upright, slowing your breathing into your own soothing breathing rhythm and bringing your warm, kind face and voice to this practice. Perhaps actually or in your mind, saying 'hello' to yourself, and 'hello' to your partner or partner's photo with the feeling of welcoming both of you here.
- Move into that part of you that has a deep commitment to be helpful and caring. That part of you that has great wisdom about human nature, how we never chose to have these emotions of sadness, grief, anger, envy, joy, nor biological motivations to connect, to find safeness, to want to avoid threat. The part of you that has developed great strength and courage through your life. Imagine moving around as this person, feeling how your body moves, how it feels, how your voice would sound if you spoke to others, the sensation of compassion, of caring, of strength, pouring out of your body and into your partner.
- Imagine looking down as if from a high-up place where you and your partner can watch what you have both been through as if watching a play or a film from a distance. You both watch with compassion, interest, curiosity about what you can see from this perspective that you might never have seen before, about yourself, about your partner, about this situation.

- You might notice your heartfelt wish that you have for both of you as you watch; what you deeply wish that both of you could know and carry with you through this experience.
- You might notice any urges you have in your body – what your body might want to do if it could.
- If you have your eyes closed, you might wish to open your eyes and look at your partner from your warm, kind, wise and strong, compassionate mind. You might wish for them to open their eyes too so you can both just sit with each other in this moment.

End of practice.

You might want to write down or share with each other what you want to remember from this:

The following can be written down individually and then shared, or just carried with you either physically or in your mind on your own.

Make a note of any difference it makes to you even if you don't share this practice with your partner.

What we have been through together/the aspects that we have shared:

What I have missed with regard to you [your partner] during this time of feeling more separate from each other:

What I am grateful and thankful for in you:

My heartfelt wish for you:

How I see our lives in the future together:

My commitment to us as a couple:

What I would like to do together

In the remainder of this day:

In the next day or so:

In the next week:

In the next month or few months:

Your notes and reflections on grief in parenthood to death losses:

Module 56: Jealousy, envy and sibling rivalry

A set of common emotions that can become heightened in the perinatal period are those to do with jealousy, envy and resentment. We can be envious of our baby's sense of freedom, ease, ability to play without worry, demand of others without shame or anxiety, and lack of responsibility, particularly if we were unable to have these experiences in our own childhood.

We might find we become jealous of our baby's delight in our partner and fear that they may come to love them more than us. We might be jealous of our partner's greeting of our baby, and perhaps even of the dog first before they greet us, or envious of our partner's ease, seeming lack of worry, and ability to calm our baby, when we feel compelled to carry a full load of worry and anxiety for our baby. Or our partner may be jealous of our close and intimate relationship with our baby which seems to get in the way of the previously intimate relationship with each other that existed before the baby.

Maybe we envy our partner's freedom to be able to complete their work before returning home, to be able to think a whole uninterrupted thought, or drink a still warm cup of coffee.

We can be jealous of our siblings who seem to be favoured by our parents in terms of child-care, time or delight in their children more than ours.

We might also be envious of other parents who have had a child without the illness, difficulty or visible difference that our baby has been born with.

And of course, we see very clearly the jealousy that can arrive when we have another baby and witness our older child struggle so much with having to share us.

These can be painful emotions, but they are entirely normal. We did not choose to have these emotions as part of our repertoire. They have been wired into us through the process of evolution. Being able to compare, judge our value in relation to others, judge whether we might be at risk of losing what is important and possibly vital to our wellbeing and survival of ourselves and our baby, could have been the difference between surviving and not surviving. So, comparison, judgement, envy and jealousy are hardwired in us and become even more fired up when we have a baby.

Indeed, with regard to sibling rivalry, for most of animal and human evolutionary history, mothers (both human and animal) had to make painful and difficult choices over which offspring to keep alive when resources were limited. Huge numbers of calories but also resources in terms of time and energy from the parents are needed to keep a child alive until they themselves can reproduce. Human mothers need the support of others, including grandmothers and their partner, in order to be able to keep all their children alive. If that support is not there then, across the course of history and described in just about every society, there is evidence that they are more likely to abandon their baby. Mostly the death of a baby in this way would not be a conscious act but would be an abandonment in the hope that somehow the baby would be taken care of by somebody else and would survive. Or the death would come about by unconscious behaviour such as giving more food or care to the more robust child without fully realising it, or 'overlaying' on the weakest or youngest baby in the night for example. This has been understood and accepted in the animal kingdom but also in human history as a very sad and regretful part of life, treated with compassion rather than shame.

This means that a strategy of fairness would have been the least favourable in terms of keeping offspring alive, as all may die. Instead 'favouritism' strategies or algorithms were favoured by evolution so that at least one child was likely to make it to reproduction. With the favouritism algorithm comes the flip side to this – that children have a wired-in 'sibling rivalry' algorithm where they are on high alert to any signs that another sibling is being favoured over them. It would literally have been a matter of life and death (and still is in countries where resources are limited, threats are high, or support is scarce). It is therefore not their fault that children will always be wanting things to be fair, or that they get profoundly jealous when another sibling comes along. It makes absolute evolutionary sense.

We also never grow out of our sibling rivalry sensitivity; even as adults, for most of human history, we were (and still are) dependent on the help from others to stay alive and healthy. And when we have our own children, we are wired to need the support of others, including our mothers, and may find our sibling rivalry algorithm coming in again if we feel our mother is spending more time caring for our sibling's children than ours. This would still stir up that ancient, evolved threat to the continuation of our genes.

So, when our baby comes along, we may find ourselves feeling childlike in our jealousy, perhaps of our baby, our partner's relationship with them, our siblings, and so on, because without realising it, this evolved sibling rivalry algorithm that was so familiar in our childhood has come alive again, bringing with it all the associated memories from our childhood.

These feelings cause us the greatest difficulty if we are not aware of them, as they can unconsciously guide our behaviour in ways which may be unhelpful, and sometimes harmful to us or to others. And if we feel ashamed of them, and become self-critical of ourselves, then we add another layer of pain to what is already there. We may end up having to engage in all sorts of safety strategies in order to avoid, block out, or manage these layers of difficult emotions or urges. None of which allow us to develop more helpful ways of coming at these experiences.

How might our compassionate self or other help us with these feelings?

- We don't need to work this out, as once we have switched systems to our compassion system, then that will work it out for us.
- So firstly, we need to switch into our compassion system: Sitting back in our seat, eyes closed or focused gently on an object, feet hip width apart on the floor. Move into a 'dignified' posture, sitting upright, bringing your shoulders up to your ears, dropping them down and back, feeling the spaciousness in your body. Bringing a warm, gentle facial expression and voice tone to your breath. Perhaps imagining greeting it; 'Hello there, breath!' Allowing your in breath, and your out breath, to begin to slow down, feeling that deep, slow, smooth rhythm of your breath. Your body might begin to feel steadier, and more stable, strong and rooted like a mighty oak tree.
- Imagine stepping into that part of yourself that has a deep commitment to being caring and compassionate as best you can. A part of you that has gathered so much wisdom over the years. A part that has great courage and strength of character.
- Or imagine that your compassionate other/image arrives and you become aware of being in the presence of the caring, kind, warm, wise, strong being who understands you inside and out.
- Imagine that your compassionate self or other looks down from above and sees you in the situation where you are feeling jealousy or envy.

What might this compassionate mind understand of this situation? What might it see? What might it say to you? How might it help you?

____

____

____

____

____

____

e.g. 'Oh, this is so hard when these feelings come upon us. They can really get in the way of what we really wish to feel, the warmth, closeness and connectedness in our relationships. This is not what you wanted to be feeling when you had your baby, was it? However, these feelings are often close by when we have relationships that are important to us, and even more so if our feelings resonate with our early or previous experiences.'

'It is not your fault that this is happening. We never chose to be able to experience such feelings, and we are also wired to be on alert to when care, resources or attention are being given to others at our expense. This is because most of our existence as humans was fraught with gathering enough resources and care to go round. Imagine our ancient lives on the African plains. If we didn't receive these resources and care, there would have been a very high risk that we would have died. Even if that is not the case now in our current situation, we still carry the wiring to alert us to the slightest danger that this might be occurring. This is not our fault.'

'Just breathe into the feelings, allow them space. Allow them to come and go, wax and wane. Hold them with your warm, kind, understanding compassionate mind. Hold them without fear or concern, but with a warm curiosity.'

Perhaps it is enough just to know that these feelings are normal. Perhaps it would help to speak to other people or read some accounts of these experiences in books or online. It might help to speak to your partner or family about this, to ask them for suggestions and help. It can also help to look at what is happening using your compassionate mind rather than your threat mind, as you may well see that what you fear is not happening at all as you see it. Our threat mind only remembers the worrying or difficult bits. That is just the nature of our threat mind.

Imagine that this jealousy or envy could be taken out of you. Perhaps we invite it to take a seat. We can regard it from our steady, wise, kind, compassionate mind and ask some questions of it with genuine curiosity and with warmth:

What might it say if we asked it how come it feels this way?

____

____

____

____

What is it like to feel this way?

____

____

____

____

When does it feel worse?

____

____

____

____

When does it feel a little better?

____

____

What is its fear for you if it were to disappear and no longer be a part of you?

How do you feel towards it as you hear these things?

How might you want to be with it?

What might you want to say to it?

How might you try and help it?

e.g. your jealous part might tell you: '*When our baby reaches out to his dad when he is in my arms I feel a kind of stab of pain in my chest. I do my best to try to hide it, but it hurts so much it almost takes my breath away. I think I am just so scared that he doesn't really love me, and that over time he will just want to be with his dad, and I will be left alone. As I am saying this, I am remembering how similar this feeling is to seeing my dad and my sister. They got on so well together and I felt so left out. It was a mixture of hurt, anxiety, anger and grief. No wonder that I am feeling this now. And I understand why I can end up trying to kind of secretly turn my baby against his dad so that he loves me more, which I have felt terrible about. But now I get why. I would love to talk to my partner about this actually and see if he can help me. I wonder if he ever feels this way too, come to think of it? He might? And perhaps others feel the same about their baby? I might have a look on some of the websites that have been so helpful so far. I bet I'm not alone with this.*'

Imagine you are a method actor who has been studying a person for many months who can bring compassion to their own jealousy and envy: how they move, how they sound if they speak, the expression on their face, how they interact with others. Now imagine stepping into this character and method acting 'as if' you are them. Notice how your body changes, your posture, how you move, how you sound, the expressions on your face, how you are in the world, how you interact with others.

How do you feel? What do you notice?

Your reflections on this section – what would you like to take hold of and remember? Anything you want to take forward from this?

When our child prefers daddy/our partner

Although some mothers might be happy or relieved for this to be the case, often this is experienced as deeply and utterly painful. Mothers describe it as a visceral experience – 'like I have been stabbed through the heart' – and it can lead to feelings of shame, self-criticism and sometimes depression.

It is considered normal for a baby to prefer mummy over daddy (or the partner in a relationship considered the 'daddy'), and it is often expected that daddy should just accept it and allow his partner to soak up her barely concealed delight. It can of course cause the father sadness and distress too, which his partner may try to rectify. But because the narrative around mothering in our society is still about the mother being the primary nurturer, in addition to the physical wound of rejection, the mother can feel a sense of shame that she is not able to do this most primal of jobs for her child.

A child preferring daddy is actually very common, and a quick internet search will reveal just how common it is. Most reassurances reiterate that this is just a phase and that, just like us as adults who might prefer one friend over another, or one relative over another and then despite it feeling intense and potentially lifelong, it switches. However, when you are in it, you have no idea whether this will be a phase, and the 'phase' could be years. So how do we manage this?

When we are hurt, we are thrown into our threat system which means we only have a specific set of options open to us; to compete, punish, shame, attack, run away. Examples of how we might be when this happens include: wanting to punish or shame our child, being angry with them, trying to put our partner down to our child, manoeuvre things so our partner ends up spending less time with our child, cling on to our child, guilt our child into being with us.

Sometimes our partner may be so hurt and mortified on our behalf that they ally with us against our child.

This is not our fault; it is just how our threat system is wired to work. But we can, with knowledge and commitment, and often some help from others, find a way of switching systems into our compassionate mind so that our threat system is no longer running the show. This then means we have a whole new set of options available to us to manage this painful situation.

Practice: Bringing the compassionate mind to the part of us that is feeling rejected by our baby

- Sit in your upright, 'dignified' posture, with your feet hip width apart and flat on the ground. Note the sensation of being in contact with the ground.
- Bring your shoulders up to your ears, then drop them down and back noting the feeling of space in your body.
- Bring your warm, kind face and warm, kind voice to your breath, perhaps imagining greeting it as if you are so pleased to have come across it, 'Hello breath!' Allow your in breath to slow down and flow deeply and smoothly into the base of your lungs. Note the pause and then feel your out breath flowing all the way out from the depth of your lungs into the air. Perhaps use your ocean breathing or toning to help lengthen the breath.
- 'Body like a mountain or an ancient oak tree, breath like the wind, mind like the wide, blue sky.'
- As your breath slows down, you might notice an increase in your sense of steadiness, or stability and sturdiness.

- Now move more fully into that part of you that has a deep commitment to caring about others including your baby. The part of you that has great strength and courage, a real willingness to step into difficult areas to make things better. A part of you that might surprise you with its courage, and its ability to keep on going, even when things get hard. You might have a sense of your wisdom, gathered over a lifetime from all your experiences, from all the people you have encountered even for the briefest of moments, from all the learning you have done as a child and as an adult. You might notice your understanding that we never chose our human brain with all our motives, emotions and behaviours. We never chose our genes or the experiences we grew up with that have contributed to the person we are today. We never chose the capacity to be jealous, to be hurt, to feel so scared of being left out or unloved. So much of what we struggle with has been shaped for us, not by us, and is not our fault. It can be very hard to be human sometimes.
- Imagine that you could look down with your warm, kind, wise, caring, strong, compassionate mind and see that part of you that is really struggling with your baby when they are showing preferences for your partner. You notice what you see, the degree of pain you are in, how this all plays out between you, your baby and your partner. You watch with warm understanding, compassion and curiosity.
- Notice how you feel towards that suffering part of you. What is your heartfelt wish for them? What would you deeply want them to know? What might you want to say to them? (Notice how your voice sounds if you speak to them, and the expression on your face.) What is your urge towards them?
- Imagine that you could swap places with them, and they could look up and see your wise, kind, understanding, strong, caring, compassionate mind looking down at them. What is it like for them to take in your heartfelt wish for them? What is it like for them to have you here with them in this way? Notice how they feel in their body as they take in your compassionate presence.
- Now imagine swapping back into your body and your compassionate mind, feeling your size, your steadiness, the spaciousness in your body. Breathing in and breathing out slowly. Getting in touch once again with your commitment to being as helpful and caring as possible, with your wisdom and strength.

- Now imagine, as you look down, that you include your struggling part, your baby and your partner in your attention. Notice how you feel towards all of them. Notice your heartfelt wish for them all. Bring your wisdom, your strength and steadiness, your kindness and understanding to all of them.

End of practice.

Write down what is coming to mind. What would you wish to share with that struggling part? What would you like her to hold on to and remember?

____

____

____

____

Who did you prefer as a child? How come? Did your preference change? When would you go to one parent and when the other?

____

____

____

____

How did you need the 'unfavoured' parent to be with you?

____

____

How is your inner critic dealing with all of this? How might you be with your inner critic? How might you help them?

What fears might this have brought up in you? How would your compassionate mind be with you and help you with these fears? See if any of these resonate with you:

(These fears are so incredibly painful. Ensure that you are still holding them with your compassionate mind:

'Body like a mountain, breath like the wind, mind like the blue sky,' warm, kind face and voice. Stepping into the part of you that has great wisdom, strength, courage and a deep commitment to being as helpful and caring as you can.)

- That you are unlovable.
- That you will be unloved.
- That your partner and baby will go off together without you, leaving you alone and abandoned.
- That you will feel ashamed in front of others.
- That you are doing something wrong.
- That you are missing out on being a proper mother. (There may be grief and loss here.)
- That you miss the cuddles and nice moments that you see your partner having with your baby and feel grief, loss or envy.

- That your child has discovered the 'real' unlovable you that you have kept hidden all these years.
- That your child has discovered that although you are not horrible, there is nothing about you that people would invest in. You are just boring, bland, uninteresting, somebody people don't even notice. (Terrifying to feel this way as for most of our evolved human life we depended on being noticed and remembered for our very survival.)
- That love is finite and there is only a set amount to go round. (This can tap into our evolved sensitivity to 'sibling rivalry' where for most of our evolved human existence a mother might have had to make difficult choices over which child to nurture and feed, if circumstances meant that she only had the resources to keep one child alive. As a consequence, we are wired to be sensitive to any hints of favouritism, even as adults, and this is not our fault.)

How might your compassionate mind help you with any memories or past experiences that have been triggered by all this (e.g. where a sibling or a friend was preferred over you, or where you felt left out or abandoned)?

How would you like to react if you could be at your compassionate best? (This shifts us out of the threat system, which can only do things like compete, be angry or punish, and instead into how we can connect with them despite them preferring daddy or our partner, for example, how to nurture our own unique relationship with our baby, what we would like to share with our baby, e.g. loving reading to them or gardening with them.)

____

____

____

____

Our compassionate mind helps to move us out of competitive mode ('Who do you love the best?') into what we deeply want for our child above all; for example, that we want to love them no matter what, even when they don't appear to love us in this way.

What do you deeply wish for your child?

____

____

____

____

Using your compassionate mind to sustain you and help you hang on in there – how might it help to sustain you whilst this is all happening?

____

____

____

____

Our compassionate mind might also help us to wonder if there is anything that we inadvertently do that might contribute to this. If we could look through the warm, understanding, wisdom and care of our compassionate mind at what is happening, what might we see? e.g. Do we have a difficult attachment relationship with our baby that we need help with? Have we been working too many hours? Do we have a stronger urge to tidy the house than be with our baby? Do we lack confidence in parenting so leave it to others? Are we not very 'fun'? Do we need to understand and accept this, or might we need help to practise being more silly and feeling more free? Perhaps we may just accept that this is something we struggle with or that it is just not something that is part of our personality, and instead we want to find a way to allow our partner and child to enjoy this aspect of their relationship?

What might you want to work on? How might your compassionate mind help you with this?

____

____

____

____

Your compassionate mind might help you to:

- Reach out to others for help, e.g. asking others, 'Can you see if I need to do anything differently? I just cannot see what it might be. I need your help here.'
- Tune in to when they *do* want you, when they do enjoy being with you. (Our threat mind will only focus on when they prefer our partner so will miss all these moments.)
- Be more at ease (so hard to do, so we really need our compassionate mind with us here), finding equanimity, holding it all more loosely even though it hurts.This looseness and ease will be picked up by our baby, helping them to feel comfortable in our company compared to when they feel the tension in us that even when things are good, we are wanting to hold on tight to them for fear this moment of connection will end.
- Move aside from the pain and jealousy and tune into the gratitude that our baby can have this wonderful relationship with our partner. That despite the deep pain of how

we feel, we can still love them. That we are doing our absolute best to mother them well even when this is happening to us.

Reflections and notes: What would you like to take hold of and remember from this section on bringing our compassionate mind to our struggles with jealousy, envy and sibling rivalry? What would you like to take forward and try? What might be your next steps?

____

____

____

____

Module 57: I don't feel anything for my baby

We discussed earlier in the book about the maternal motivational system or network in a mother's brain that appears to become switched on and turned up during pregnancy. It is thought these changes occur to promote bonding, and sensitive, attuned interactions with our baby. However, there are many instances and examples where this maternal motivational system isn't so powerfully turned up, or gets turned down or off altogether. We understand this very well in the animal kingdom. So, we know that female sheep (ewes) need to feel calm and looked after when they are pregnant, birthing or nursing their young. They need to smell their lamb very quickly after birth and to have the opportunity to lick and make physical contact with it to bond. We know that some ewes are much more maternal than others and we may never know why, but we accept that without judgement. We know that animal parents with more than one offspring might give up on the smallest, weakest or sickest, and that they might stand by and watch whilst bigger offspring attack and eventually kill the weakest one. It is understood that it takes such a lot of resources to raise offspring until they can reproduce, that when there is very little food, when healthier offspring might be put at risk if the weakest was given a share of limited resources, if the mother is weak or ill herself, when a species that relies on support in caring for the offspring does not have that support, then an animal mother may abandon her baby.

The maternal network in a human mother's brain can, it seems, be turned up, down or even off in similar circumstances. Indeed, all over the world, still today, and certainly for most of human history, babies would be consciously or unconsciously left to die or be killed. The reasons are similar to the rest of the animal kingdom and include: where there are too few resources to go round, where there is so little support that it overwhelms the resources the parents have, where there is so much threat in the parents' lives that it is hard to keep themselves safe as well as a baby, when the baby looks like they might not survive, when a mother has had a pregnancy and/or birth that has depleted or harmed her to such a degree that she doesn't have the resources within herself to parent the baby at that time.

Since the advent of birth control, higher standards of living, and greater understanding and awareness, abandoning or killing a baby is incredibly rare, and thankfully there are considerable resources in many countries to help support parents, but it still does happen. Because of this it is crucial that women feel they can come forward for help rather than be kept quiet through shame. There are many different kinds of help which can bring online or turn up a warm, connected relationship with our baby. (If you are worried you might harm your baby, call people you feel will support you straight away and contact your GP, your midwife or health visitor, or Accident and Emergency if you are very worried – there is help available for you, and the aim will be to help you through this *with* your baby unless you decide that your baby temporarily or perhaps permanently should be looked after by somebody else.) Feeling like you are not connected to your baby, wishing you hadn't had your baby or both loving and hating your baby are very common.

There are many reasons for this, and sometimes we need the help of specialist services to discover why, or indeed we may never find out.

But both with and without help these difficult feelings usually pass. Whilst we are struggling in it though, this can be hard to believe. If we can understand that we didn't choose for it to be this way, that this is not our fault, and that we are doing our best to try to improve the situation, then we can get through it step by step. But it can be very hard, especially on our own, so getting support of family, friends and specialist services can be vital, and there are many incredible treatments that can help, and can help surprisingly quickly in many cases.

Some of the reasons why we might find it hard to connect with, or love, or want to be with our baby include:

- Pre- or postnatal depression – this affects all of our motivational systems including the maternal one.
- A difficult pregnancy or birth.
- Where the baby appears ill or disfigured.
- A lack of support.
- Chronic stress.
- When having a baby overwhelms our internal and/or external resources.
- Where the baby becomes connected to threat or harm, for example when it becomes linked to severe morning sickness or a scary or traumatic birth.
- Where the baby triggers difficult memories from the past, for example, having

responsibility to care for parents or siblings when you were a child yourself, traumatic experiences or difficult attachment experiences.

- When the baby is not sending out care-receiving signals, for example if the baby is ill, very pre-term, or is neurodivergent in some way.
- Where you find it hard to understand your baby's cues.
- Where you and your baby have different personality traits to each other, e.g. one of you is more introverted and the other more extroverted.
- Where the mother and baby are separated such as when the mother and/or baby are ill and are being cared for in different places.
- When the baby is regularly and chronically distressed, for example, when experiencing colic or difficulty feeding.
- D-MER (Dysphoric Milk Ejection Reflex) – where the hormone involved with the let-down reflex in breastfeeding causes temporary feelings of anxiety, dread, irritability, sadness and tearfulness.

There are many more reasons. Often finding out why can take away shame, guilt and anxiety. There are also many ways to help parents feel connected to their babies, and in many cases, this can happen quite quickly despite it often feeling quite hopeless. So do seek help.

Here are some ways that have helped mothers to spark feelings of love and connection for their baby:

- 'Watch Me Play' (ask your health visitor about this. Detailed guidance is also available on the internet): Follow baby's lead. Give baby space to send out initiatives to you, then you receive it and send back a response, e.g. copying and adding something, then give space for baby to respond.
- Slow things down: A common response when anxious is to be intrusive rather than being led by baby, so slow down your breathing and just become curious and interested in the baby – getting out of your own head ('*I'm no good at this. I am boring, I have no idea what to do next*) and into your baby's head. Taking pressure off yourself and just aiming to be interested in what they are doing – 'Watch, Wait and Wonder'.
- Grandparents' sites, e.g. Gransnet: These have ideas that you can have on hand so you can scaffold yourself and give yourself a secure base from which to then be slow and curious with baby.

- Connect face to face: This synchronises our brain waves and our oxytocin with our baby.
- Move to physical closeness and touch where possible: This triggers oxytocin, the hormone involved in connection.
- Work out enjoyable contact for yourself as well as baby: For example, massaging hand cream into baby's hand, having made sure you have told baby what you are doing and allowed baby time to prepare. Only do this if they seem happy for this to happen.
- Holding baby in a soft sleepsuit.
- Oxygen mask: Making sure you feel safe, soothed and looked after before you try to connect with your baby, perhaps by doing one of the compassionate mind practices first.
- Not worrying about your feelings at the moment: Focus your motivational system of compassion (motivational systems still work without the emotions that go with them although it is much harder) – to be helpful, to be caring, whilst appreciating the courage it takes to be working on this because it is important to you and your baby.
- Notice your environment: Try moving to one that you enjoy being in yourself and be with your baby in that one (one mum couldn't quite believe that she began to feel some sparks of warmth for her baby when she bought some furry cushions and a soft blanket for her lovely, minimalist but rather cold and sparse front room). See if being outside in nature makes things easier rather than being inside, for example.
- Sometimes we try so hard that we end up in our threat system rather than our soothing system, so just give it all a light touch. It is like making a spark for a fire; we can end up blowing on it too hard and then accidentally blow it out, so just be gentle with yourself – it is the keeping on facing in the direction of your baby rather than worrying about the feelings that is the key. The feelings will come.
- Video interaction guidance (VIG) principles: this is an intervention where an interaction is videoed (for example between a mother and her baby) by a VIG-trained professional. The VIG professional then picks out stills or clips of instances of connection (or whatever the mother would like to try to do more of) and plays them back to the mother the next time they meet. VIG can work very rapidly because, unlike VIG,

our threat minds don't see what we are actually doing right, only what we are doing wrong.

We don't want to be relying on our critic or threat mind to tell us how it is going – it will only see all the times it didn't go well, and you can see those well enough for yourself. Instead we need to come from the compassion system to capture what is going well and this then allows us to also see what to do more of. VIG is great for this.

It also captures the essence of what works with our children too. Because of our human wiring we will react strongly to what we *don't* want them to do so they learn this really well. We can end up inadvertently adding feelings of anger, anxiety, shame and so on to our children too when we tell them off for example. Often, we forget to help and reward them with what they did right and what went well, despite our best intentions.

We need to use the principles of VIG for this too. In other words, to shine a light on what they do well, or what is going in the right direction even if it's only by one degree – '*I saw you try really hard not to take that toy off of your little sister. That was good.*'

The same for us – it doesn't need to be the number ten (the most difficult) on our ladder of achievement – number one is the first step in the right direction (or number 0.5 if number one turned out to be too high a step to reach yet).

- What most people wanted from their parents wasn't necessarily the most perfectly nurturing of environments, but an awareness that their parents held them in mind and really tried to do their best because they cared about their children. It is the holding in mind, the caring motivation to be 'helpful and not harmful' as best we can, and that if, and when, we do mess up, we feel guilty rather than ashamed and are moved to say sorry and to try to do it better, that is important.
- Notice what helps you to be in your soothing/safeness system – this is the system of connection. See if you can find ways to connect this to times when you are with your baby, so you develop an association between them and feelings of soothing and safeness.
- Be with people who will support and help you rather than take over looking after the baby – be clear to them, and yourself, that although a bit of a break might help you to move from threat to soothing, letting them take over fully might be a safety strategy coming from your threat system rather than your compassionate mind. Consider what a compassionate mind might think would be the best way for this person to help you with your bond with your baby.

- Be with yourself too rather than leaving yourself alone – be your own best encourager and supporter. Use your compassionate self or compassionate image for this.
- Try the compassionate / safe / your place practice with the intention of bringing your baby there to see how this place might help you both.
- Share the care of your baby – they want quite basic needs from their parents. For most of our evolutionary lives there would have been plenty of other people on hand desperate to play with our baby, cuddle them, show them things – a whole village of people – you don't need to be, and can't be, an entire village for them, not even you and your partner are enough; let 'the village' help.
- Compassionate letter writing to yourself, and to you and your baby.
- Baby massage.
- Singing with your baby.
- Dancing gently with your baby.
- Joint activities with your baby.
- Playing musical instruments together.
- Painting jointly with your baby.
- 'Circle of security', which teaches how to be a secure base and safe haven for your baby. It gives clear direction which helps to 'scaffold' the development of connection with your baby (ask your health visitor about this).
- Support e.g. family, Homestart.
- Being resourced and nourished yourself.
- Being rehoused.
- Help with your other children.
- Neurodiversity support and support groups.
- Learning to read, write, do mathematics, so that you feel ready rather than anxious about sharing these with your child.
- EMDR (eye movement desensitisation and reprocessing) for trauma including birth trauma (speak to your health visitor or GP about this).

Reflections and notes: What would you like to take hold of and remember from this section on bringing our compassionate mind to when we don't feel anything for our baby? What would you like to take forward and try? What might be your next steps?

___

___

___

___

Module 58: 'Arrested anger' and 'arrested escape' in motherhood

As we have seen throughout this book, we have evolved defences to enable us to deal with threat and to return to a state of safeness. These evolved defences in humans include being able to push away or confront (anger–fight) or to escape, run away or avoid (flight). When these natural defences are thwarted or blocked ('arrested') then we can move to a state of panic and helplessness, feeling trapped and powerless in a difficult situation. Research based on interviews with people who attended an emergency department following incidents of self-harm and suicidal intent found that just before the self-harm incident, feelings of entrapment (wanting to get away from things but being unable to) and of arrested anger (feeling angry with somebody but being unable to tell them) were very high.

Motherhood can sometimes create circumstances where feelings of both entrapment and arrested anger arise together. In motherhood, what we are trying to get away from may be external to us; for example, becoming a mother, our baby, our partner. Or it may be inside of us; for example, our self-critic, or unpleasant or scary feelings. As discussed earlier, being unable to express anger may arise from a whole constellation of issues including being female in a society where a female should not be angry, issues to do with being a mother, our own history, or our partner.

It is tragic, but therefore not surprising, that when both arrested escape and thwarted anger come together for a mother, she may feel the only way out is to self-harm or to take her own life or the life of her baby (or both). Although carrying this out is exceedingly rare, suicidal thoughts and attempts after having a baby are not unheard of, so being able to bring this into the open is crucial in being able to offer help. When our minds have moved into this degree of threat they can only see one solution. Once we can move into a different state through feeling safe, all sorts of other solutions arise that we could not see before.

Interestingly, the process of being asked about their experiences of self-harm actually helped participants in the research to make sense of their feelings, to be able to put them into words, to feel empowered, validated, and to have a deeper insight into their own situation. This ended up reducing their shame and self-criticism even though this wasn't the primary intention of the interviews. So, despite nothing changing at that point in their circumstances (they had merely answered the questions whilst in the emergency department) they felt significantly better. This demonstrates the power of talking about and understanding our emotions, even when our threat mind and self-critic is telling us that simply talking about it could never possibly make a difference in the face of such extreme feelings. The message, as ever, is to reach out, to your midwife, health visitor, GP, emergency department, calling '999' in the UK if you feel you cannot keep yourself or your baby safe, who are all trained to look out for these very experiences in new mothers, and to trusted friends and relatives. There are mother-and-baby units and other services set up for situations precisely like these.

Reflections and notes: What would you like to take hold of and remember from this section on bringing our compassionate mind to arrested anger and arrested escape in the context of motherhood. What would you like to take forward and try? What might be your next steps?

____

____

____

____

Module 59: Practices and exercises to help with difficult thoughts and emotions in motherhood

Exercise: Finding the wisdom in our difficult thoughts and feelings

- Sit in your 'dignified' posture, upright, with your head up, shoulders back and down, feet hip width apart and in contact with the ground. Bring your warm, kind face and voice to your breath, perhaps imagining greeting it with delight and gratitude for just being here supporting you, steadying you in the background, day and night ('Hello breath!').
- Allow your breathing to become deep, slow and smooth, and to settle into its own soothing rhythm. As it does you might notice an increase in the sense of stability and steadiness in your body. Notice how you might move and walk and interact with people from this place of steadiness, strength and calm. Your sense of being as strong as a mighty oak tree but able to bend and move with all that life may throw at you, coming back to that place of steadiness each time.
- Allow yourself to move into that part of you that has great wisdom, that understands our difficult human minds; that we never chose to have these emotions as part of us, that we never chose to be able to think these thoughts or to have the experiences and genes that have shaped us through our lives. Notice the amount of wisdom that you have acquired throughout your life, from all the teaching and training you have done, from all the things you have read and watched on the TV, from all the people you have encountered in your life. Move into that part that also has a deep commitment to being as caring and helpful as possible, even when it is so hard to do so. That part that has a strength and courage that perhaps even surprises you – that has meant you have shown up and done some very difficult things.
- Imagine that your difficult thought or feeling that you want help with could be taken out of you and seated on a chair. From your place of steady, wise, strong, kind compassion, just sit with it, with kindness, interest and curiosity. Nothing to do but to get to know it a little. To see what it has to say. To see what you might discover from talking with it in this way.
- If this feels too hard to do, imagine your compassionate other/being is here and will be sitting, talking to this difficult thought or feeling instead of you. You will just be listening in and watching from another room.

You might want to find out (see if you can answer any of these questions yourself):

When it first arrived in you

____

____

____

What triggered it

____

____

____

What it was really struggling with about this

____

____

____

What it really wants you to know and understand about what it is struggling with

____

____

____

What else it might be feeling or thinking about this

What it might fear if it were no longer able to be part of your life, or if for some reason it had gone off for a wander when you needed it

Ways it might be trying to help you, albeit from the only thing it has access to – your threat system

What might really help it to settle

- If you feel pulled into the emotions or thoughts of this part, or begin to feel anxious, overwhelmed or angry, then just anchor back into your compassionate mind – your 'dignified' posture, your slow, steady breathing, your wisdom, your strength, your motivation to be as caring and helpful as you can. Feel your body growing in size and spaciousness, steadying and becoming more stable once again, then return back to this part, with nothing to do but carry out this interview, with curiosity, interest, warmth and non-judgement.

- When you are ready to finish, just bring your attention back to the sounds in this room, allowing them in through your ears. Notice the feel of the chair supporting you, of your feet in contact with the ground, and your hands in your lap – perhaps wiggling them. When you are ready, open your eyes. You might want to stretch and move.

What reflections do you have from this exercise? What do you want to hold onto and remember from this exercise?

____

____

____

____

____

____

Practice: 'Leaves in the stream' – mindfulness to thoughts

- Sit with your eyes closed or gaze settled gently on an object. Have your feet hip width apart, in contact with the ground. Your body upright in its 'dignified' posture, back straight, head up, shoulders brought up to your ears then dropped back and down, allowing your body to feel spaciousness, steady and strong.
- Bring your warm, kind face and voice to your breath, perhaps imagining greeting it with warmth and gratitude ('Hello breath!'). Allow your in breath to slow down and deepen then really slow down your out breath, letting it become smooth, gentle and slow. Begin to feel the soothing rhythm of your breath. As you do so, you might notice the feeling of your body becoming a little steadier, a little sturdier and more stable.

- Imagine now that you find yourself sitting comfortably by a beautiful stream. The sun feels just right on your skin and creates sparkles on the water. You can hear the sound of the water just babbling, gurgling and moving along. You might hear the sound of birds and of a gentle breeze rustling the leaves of nearby trees. You might notice the smells, perhaps of the grass or the trees. You feel settled, calm and steady and are enjoying sitting here with nothing to do but sit by the stream.
- Imagine now that each thought you have, appears written on a leaf that floats, bobs and twirls gently down the stream. The next thought you have gently bobs past you on its leaf. You just watch calmly as each thought moves past you. At first you might think that you are not having any thoughts – this in itself is a thought. Just allow it to appear on a leaf and watch it float down the stream. You might think that you aren't doing it right, or that it is hard, or that you keep forgetting to put a thought on a leaf. These are all thoughts. Allow each one to float on past on its leaf.
- Your mind will wander, as all minds do. Each time you notice this just gently guide it back to the leaves in the stream.
- After a while you might start to notice how it feels in your body to be able to watch the thoughts floating past, and how this compares to when you get caught up in your thoughts.
- Often people notice a calmness when watching the thoughts compared to feeling more anxious or wound up when they get caught up in their thoughts. Don't worry about what you notice or don't notice though; just keep coming back to the leaves in the stream. Allowing each thought to arise, appear on the leaf, then drift away. Nothing more to do.
- Just notice if there are some thoughts that you feel you want to take hold of and not let drift away, and others that you want to hurry along. Simply notice these urges with a gentle nod, and let them go. If they appear as thoughts, then, again, put these thoughts onto the leaves and let them drift along too.
- If it feels hard to do, particularly if you find yourself moving into the story of your thoughts or getting upset by them, then toning has been found to be very helpful. This is where you accompany your mindfulness with a deep, long 'ou' (as in 'moo') sound

that you can feel resonating in your chest. It can help to place your hand on your chest so you can feel the vibration. Just keep repeating the sound, making it as long as you can. It has been found to be very calming and helps to regulate your heart and breathing rate whilst doing mindfulness practices, particularly for difficult thoughts and emotions.

- Stay here by the stream for as long as you wish.
- When you are ready, bring your attention to the sounds in your room, allowing them in through your ears. Notice the feel of the chair underneath you, supporting you. Notice the feel of your feet in contact with the floor and your hands in your lap, perhaps moving them. When you are ready, gently open your eyes. You might want to stretch and move. See if you can take this calm, mindful manner with you into the next part of your day.

End of practice.

What did you notice from this practice? What would you like to take hold of and remember?

____

____

____

____

Practice: Compassion to having difficult thoughts and feelings

- Sit with your eyes closed or your gaze gently resting on an object in your 'dignified' posture with your back and head upright, feet hip width apart and in contact with the ground. Lift your shoulders up to your ears, drop them back and down, feeling the increase in space and openness in your chest.
- Bring your warm, kind face and voice to your breath, perhaps greeting it as if you have just encountered someone or something that is dear to you, perhaps a person or an animal, or a favourite tree or plant – 'Hello breath!' Allow your in breath to slow down, feel the pause, then allow your out breath to flow smoothly and gently all the way from the base of your lungs, up and out into the air. Notice your breathing beginning to find its own soothing rhythm, slow, smooth, gentle, like a breeze through the trees.
- Imagine that you notice a compassionate being appearing near to you. It may be the compassionate part of you that is committed to being as caring and helpful as it can, the part of you that is wise, strong and courageous. Or it may be another being that has turned up for you, to help you. You sense its deep compassion; its warmth and kindness, its wisdom – it may have been around for many years, perhaps hundreds of years, and understand all the struggles that humans ever go through. You are aware of its strength and the feeling that it could bear whatever life, and you, might throw at it. That it stays steady, strong, understanding, wise and compassionate. You sense that it knows you inside and out; there is nothing you need to tell it, or reveal to it, it knows you deeply. It has seen you go through your current life, and has seen all the way back through the generations. It knows just how come you are struggling so much with your feelings of becoming a mother and towards your baby. It is here to help you, support you, be with you, with kindness, warmth and understanding.
- You notice its appearance; whether it is more of a sense of a mist or a light or whether it has a shape or a body. It may be human, or an animal, or perhaps a tree or mountain. Is it male or female, genderless, both? If it speaks, notice the tone of its voice. If it has a face, notice the expression on its face. Notice how it moves.

- How does it relate to you? It knows just what you need. It may just be a presence standing nearby, or perhaps it sits near or with you. It may just rest a hand on your arm or wrap itself around you, or hold you. It is here for you, forever. It will never leave you. This is your compassionate being. Whatever it does, you feel yourself allowing its presence, even if this is tentatively so, beginning to be able to breath out, to calm, to feel relief, to feel tension beginning to flow out of you.
- You become aware of its heartfelt wish for you. It may speak. Hear and take in what it says. Notice how it feels to hear those words. It may give you a gift. Take the gift and notice how it feels to have it.
- Notice how it feels in your body to have this compassionate being here with you, for you.
- When you are ready, bring your attention to the sounds in your room, to the chair supporting you, to your feet and your hand, perhaps moving them. When you are ready, gently open your eyes. You might wish to stretch and move. Take this feeling with you as best you can into the next part of your day.

End of practice.

Your reflections on this practice: What do you want to hold onto and take with you from this practice. What do you want to remember?

____

____

____

____

Exercise: Compassionate letter writing for difficult thoughts and emotions

(See section on compassionate letter writing for a more detailed description.)

When you are experiencing really challenging feelings and thoughts, something that feels more substantial and real can sometimes be more helpful than imagery work. Writing a letter to yourself grounds you to your pen and to the paper. As always, do your compassionate mind practice first to ensure you are writing from the compassionate part, whether it is that part of yourself, or a compassionate other. Once you have done your practice, allow your compassionate other or self to pick up your pen and write. See what it writes. This letter is supportive, kind, warm, wise, non-judgemental and expresses its understanding of just how much you are suffering right now.

A compassionate letter to yourself:

Dear [your name]

____

____

____

____

____

____

____

____

____

____

____

____

____

When you have written it, read it through slowly and with warmth, as if that warm, kind, compassionate being is reading it to you.

You might wish to keep or discard the letter, whatever is most helpful to you.

Your reflections on this exercise. What do you want to take note of and remember?

A compassionate letter to you and your baby

You might wish to write a letter to yourself and your baby from your compassionate other or being. Even though this is likely to be hard to do, it can be very powerful. As always, start with your compassionate mind practice of compassionate self or compassionate other to ensure this is written from your compassionate mind.

Your compassionate being sees just how hard this all is for both of you. It also sees, despite the struggles, all the aspects that connect you, what you have both been through, and how to help both of you with all of this. It expresses its understanding of just how this has come about, and that this is nobody's fault, just a coming together of a whole series of events, biology, history, genes, current circumstance. It is supportive, warm, wise, kind, understanding, non-judgemental and compassionate.

Dear [your name] and [your baby's name]

When you have finished writing your letter, read it through slowly, with a warm voice, as if your compassionate being is reading it to you and your baby.

You might want to keep this letter or discard it. Whatever is most helpful to you.

Your reflections on this exercise. What do you want to take note of and remember?

Reflections and notes: What would you like to take hold of and remember from this section of practices and an exercise to help with the difficult thoughts and emotions of motherhood? What would you like to take forward and try? What might be your next steps?

SECTION 9:

Looking forward: Resources for continuing to build a compassionate life

This section is about what will help us to continue our compassionate mind journey. As we have seen, our minds are wired to be easily overtaken by threat. It takes a great deal of work and practice to be able to create our compassionate mind as a pattern that we can move into easily. Our lives will be a constant process of getting caught in threat, realising we have been, then trying to get back to our compassionate mind. Sometimes we may have long periods where we forget all about our compassionate mind.

This section includes some resources that might help you to get back to your compassionate mind. It is also your place to collect together anything that you have found helpful throughout this book that you want to be able to find quickly. These might also include other resources such as postcards, sayings, titles of songs, ideas, titles of films or books, anything at all that you have come across outside of this book that you have found helpful to build and maintain your compassionate mind. (See https://overcoming.co.uk/715/resources-to-download for downloadable resources that you might want to add here.)

Module 60: Reflections on where I am now and where I hope to be heading

We have covered a great deal in this book. All the way from how we arrive here with brains, emotions, genes and experiences that we have not chosen but which shape profoundly how we live our lives. Through why compassion is so important to us and how we can lay the foundations for creating a compassionate mind, not just in ourselves but also in our baby and maybe even others too. Then to building and deepening our compassionate mind. And finally, to putting our compassionate mind to work in some easier and some very difficult areas of our lives.

It will have taken you a great deal of commitment to get to this stage of the book, but also real strength of character and courage. Particularly as some of what we have covered here is about our deepest struggles and suffering. Hopefully, it has increased your wisdom too. This workbook really has required your compassionate mind.

What are some of the learning points that you have found particularly helpful in this workbook?

____

____

____

____

____

____

What would you want to pass on from this workbook to someone who is entering motherhood?

What would you want to pass on to your baby from this workbook?

What do you want to pass on to your partner?

What have you noticed you might be doing a little differently as a result of your work with this book? (Remember to look at this through the eyes of your compassionate mind.)

____

____

____

____

____

____

What changes do you think you partner might have noticed in you as you worked through this book?

____

____

____

____

____

____

What changes do you think your baby might have noticed in you as you worked through this book?

____

____

____

____

Where would you like to go from here?

What will help you with this?

What might help you with this on a daily basis?

What will help you put this into place and keep it going?

What might help you with this on a weekly or monthly basis?

What might help you put this into place and keep it going?

How will your compassionate mind help you with the inevitable setbacks to these plans?

What will you take from your work with this book to help you get through the inevitable tough times of life?

The following practice is one that many have really enjoyed doing. It can have a real impact in terms of helping us to become more consciously aware of, and then move towards, the life that we would like to lead.

Practice: A day in the life of me at my compassionate best

- You will need some paper and a pen for this, or you can just do this in your imagination. Writing it down can be powerful and helpful. (This exercise can be downloaded from https://overcoming.co.uk/715/resources-to-download)
- Sit in your 'dignified' posture, your back and head upright, your feet hip width apart and in contact with the floor – feeling grounded. Bring your shoulders up to your ears, drop them back and down. Notice the feeling of an increase in space and openness in your body.
- Bring your warm kind face and your warm kind voice to your breath – perhaps greeting it with warmth and maybe gratitude for all it does for you. Allow your in breath to slow down. Notice the pause and then allow your out breath to flow all the way out, gently and smoothly. Allow your body and your breath to continue slowing down until you feel your breath finding its own soothing rhythm. As it does so, you might notice the feel of your body increasing in steadiness and stability.
- Move into that part of you that is really committed to being as helpful and compassionate as you can. That part of you with great wisdom that understands the difficult and amazing human brain that we have that we didn't choose, and how we are shaped by our genes, and our background which we didn't choose either. The wisdom you have acquired through all your experiences and from the people you have encountered on the way who have all contributed to your knowledge in one way or another. Notice your sense of strength and courage – that part of you that has helped you to do and get through some difficult things in your life.
- Now imagine rolling time forward to arrive at a point where you find yourself at your compassionate best. (This may be a few years in the future, many years in the future or hundreds of years in the future if this frees you up to imagine this.) You might notice how old you are: ______________________

End of practice.

Now allow your compassionate self to pick up the pen and write a diary entry for your day.

Where do you wake up? Are you in a house or another kind of dwelling? A campervan? A tent? Where are you?

____

____

____

____

____

Notice what your room is like, what your surroundings are like in this place that you are in. How is it decorated? What colours have been used? What materials have been used? It is a joy to wake up here.

____

____

____

____

____

Notice your bed and the feel of your sheets and how wonderful they feel to you. Become aware of the light and the shade and the time of the day and the season you are in. What is your bed like? What time of the day or night is it? What season are you in?

____

____

____

You might notice how you feel inside as you wake up. You might notice a sense of joy, perhaps of playfulness, of energy. Perhaps you feel settled, calm, peaceful. You might have a sense of being able to really breathe out, of feeling free and at ease. How do you feel?

Get up and have a look outside. What is the view? What can you see? Notice the colours, the light and the shade. How far can you see? What do you see to the left and the right of you?

Become aware of whether there is anybody else in this place with you. If so, become aware of where they are. Inside? Outside? Gone out for a while or for the day?

Are there any animals or pets here with you?

What do you do next? What does the next part of your day look like?

Write down your plan for today.

How will your evening be?

How will your night-time be?

Is this a typical day? What do you do on other days?

____

____

____

____

____

The more detail we can put in, the clearer our values become to us, and the more likely we are to consciously or unconsciously begin to make our diary entry become more of a reality.

Reflections from this exercise. What was this like to do? What would you like to hold onto and remember from this?

____

____

____

____

____

Module 61: My resources for supporting and sustaining my compassionate mind

My compassionate letter to myself:

Stick this in here from the compassionate letter writing section so that you can read it whenever you need to. (Compassionate letter templates can be downloaded from https://overcoming.co.uk/715/resources-to-download) You might also want to post it to yourself or leave a copy somewhere where you will come across it at a later date, for example in your Christmas decorations box – this is very powerful as it feels like somebody else has written it to you.

My compassionate letters to others:

(This might be to your baby, to your partner, a parent, you and your baby – whoever it is helpful to write to. You might want to give it to them, or just keep it here or write it then rip it up. Whatever is helpful. Don't forget to read through the compassionate letter writing section first.)

My formulation:

Write down or stick in your formulation from the formulation section here so that you have it as a reminder. (You can download the formulation sheet from https://overcoming.co.uk/715/resources-to-download)

Or you might want to just write down what particularly struck you about your formulation and what you want to remember from it.

Module 62: Remember this: Phrases to help guide us when we get a little lost

No matter how long you have been practising the compassionate mind approach, the design of the threat mind means we will still end up falling in the 'threat' river over and over again. But the more we practise the less we fall in, and when we do fall in, we notice and can get out again more and more quickly. So, falling into the threat mind is normal, no matter how much work we've done on this. In fact, working on our compassionate mind is a life's work. The most important thing is, if we fall in the threat 'river' 100 times, we get out 100 times.

It is helpful to have ways of reminding ourselves how to get back on track again; we can imagine them as lighthouses that guide us back to the path when we have wandered off. These are some reminders that people have found helpful over the years:

1. ***'To be helpful and not harmful.'***

   Paul Gilbert's definition of compassion. Useful as a quick check in the moment when we are not sure if what we are about to do or think is compassionate.

2. ***Change your body to change your mind.***

   By changing our posture, our breathing, our facial expression and our voice tone, even the way we move, we change the way we think and even the memories we have access to.

3. ***Our internal relationships operate the same as external ones.***

   We have the same brain and body set-up to deal with relationships with real people as we do for relationships with ourselves. This is why our self-critic can be so powerful and harmful to us. It is also why developing a compassionate self or imaginary compassionate other/being works.

4. ***Remember to switch systems.***

   Our threat system will take hold of us easily. This is the way it is designed. If we try to think or act without switching to the system of the compassionate mind, then our thoughts, actions, memories, even the decision to try a compassionate mind practice, will be governed by the threat system.

5. ***Even when your threat system tells you that doing a compassionate mind practice is pointless, do it anyway.***

   This is what the threat system *will* say. So, we need to switch systems into our compassionate mind even when (or especially when) our threat system provides a seemingly convincing argument against it.

6. ***Remember the third chair.***

   When we think about the parts or patterns of ourselves, we have our self-critic who sits in the first chair and the submissive or beaten-down part in the second chair who listens to the critic. The submissive part cannot change the mind of the self-critic or defend itself as it is the submissive part. Therefore, we need the compassionate mind to step in (the third chair). They bring their wisdom, support, strength, care and encouragement to the second chair (the anxious, submissive part) but they also bring it to the critic (first chair) to help identify the fear that drives the critic and how to help to settle it.

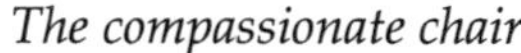

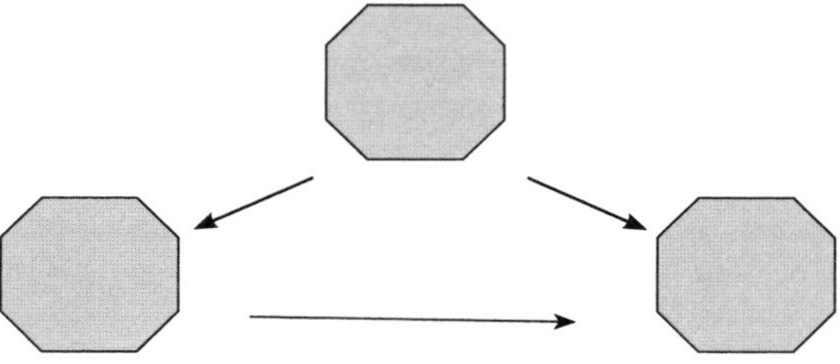

The self-critic's chair *The submissive part's chair*

7. ***Acting 'as if'.***

We don't need to try to force ourselves into believing we are the compassionate self or compassionate other. Instead, we can unhook ourselves from beliefs that might limit us by saying to ourselves – 'I know I am not . . . (e.g. compassionate) but what might I do/say/think if I were?'

8. ***Mindfulness is moving into the part of our mind that is like the clear blue sky. Everything else is the clouds.***

   We can observe without judgement, any aspect including our thoughts, feelings, body sensations, interactions with others, memories, sounds, etc. We can see that these all just pass through us like weather patterns.

9. ***'Body like a mountain, breath like the wind, mind like the clear blue sky.'***

   The start of any of our practices, reminding us to change our posture and our breath and to bring in our mindfulness.

10. ***A warm, kind face and a warm, kind voice.***

    The part we always add to 'Body like a mountain, breath like the wind, mind like the clear blue sky'. Together these form the foundation of all our work where we are 'changing the body to change the mind' ('switching systems').

11. ***Remember to switch to reading words or saying thoughts back to yourself with a warm, slow voice and facial expression.***

    Even when we have done a practice to write a compassionate letter, or we have generated compassionate alternatives to critical thinking, we can still read them back with a slightly cold or matter-of-fact voice. Changing deliberately to a warm, very slowed down, voice and face can be powerful and be the difference between shrugging off the words or enabling them to sink in and actually change our brain and our memories.

12. ***It's not your fault.***

    So much of who we are and how we struggle is to do with how our brains have evolved over millions of years, the genes that we have and the experiences that really shaped us as we grew up, none of which we chose.

13. ***But it is your responsibility.***

    Although we never chose any of this, this is the mind, body, genes, emotions and so on that we have, so it is up to us to work out how to manage ourselves the best we can. Like if somebody bumped into us and knocked us over in the street. This is not our fault. But then ultimately it is down to us to work out what to do about it rather than just staying on the floor.

14. ***Our baby as our teacher.***

When we struggle, it can help to come back to our baby, as they really show us our old brain and how humans are set up, before their new brain comes in to make them self-conscious and it all becomes more complicated. They can help us to see that these struggles are really not our fault.

15. ***Notice the 'dance' of your safety strategies in your life.***

We develop conscious and unconscious ways of keeping ourselves safe even as babies. These are not our fault. They may carry on into adulthood and to times and places even when we are now safe and don't need them anymore. This is not our fault either, as we have also evolved to have the strategy of 'better safe than sorry'. We can however use our compassionate mind to help us to notice with warm curiosity when this dance happens and ultimately to help us to develop a new 'dance' that fits our new life.

16. ***Bring your compassionate mind rather than your threat system to your critic.***

Our internal relationships work the same as external ones. If we try to destroy, cast out, humiliate or attack our self-critic it will just react the same as a critical person outside of us would. Instead, we need to bring the strength, wisdom, intention to be helpful and not harmful of our compassionate mind to the self-critic to see what drives it (usually fear) and how to help it.

17. ***Remember to 'complete the triangle' when experiencing strong emotions.***

i. e.g. grief in self/other

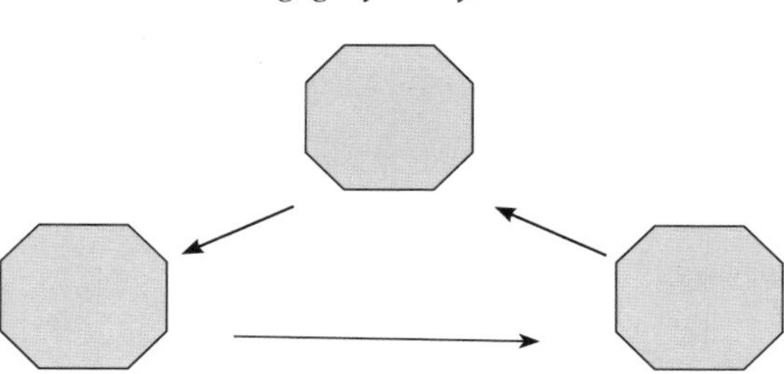

ii. Do compassionate self/other practice *iii. Relate to grief from compassionate self/other*

When we feel strong emotions, they can seem to engulf us. They will govern our actions and thoughts. We can 'switch systems', into our compassionate self or compassionate other (which is not easy to start with when we are in the midst of strong emotions but gets easier as the practice progresses). But we don't 'leave the emotion behind', instead we then turn back towards it, but now from the position of our compassionate mind, and simply relate to it from this place.

18. ***Many circumstances make being compassionate much harder.***

When we are tired, in a hurry, in pain, worried, then these make even the most compassionate person struggle to be compassionate. It is not our fault, just the power of the threat system.

19. ***Remember to 'turn on the light and look for the door'.***

The nature of attention means that whatever we focus on seems to 'light up' and become bigger in our awareness. The rest fades into the shadows. But just because it is in shadow doesn't mean it has gone completely. When we are in threat, or our self-critic has hold of us, it doesn't mean our compassionate self has gone – we just need to shift our attention to find it again. So, we need to 'switch on the light and look for the door' that takes us into the room where our compassionate self or compassionate other was all along ('switch systems' – do the practice).

20. ***We never chose the beginning of our story, but we can choose to change it a word at a time from now on.***

By practising and understanding and relating to ourselves in more compassionate ways, we are changing our very biology and brain. We can take control of how we want to be able to relate to others and ourselves from now on. (Not totally, but we may have more control and influence than we imagined.)

21. ***What fires together, wires together.***

The idea of neuroplasticity. We can create new brain connections by thinking, acting, feeling in different ways.

22. ***Learn in the shallow end, not the deep end.***

When we are trying to master something new, start when it's easiest and work up towards the hardest element, the same way we would help our baby learn something new. It may seem obvious, but as humans we only tend to try new things when we need them – this is usually when we have 'fallen in the deep end'. So, we need to be learning new skills even when we don't need them in that moment, which is often hard for humans to be motivated to do.

23. ***It is not just the absence of threat; we also need to detect safeness, to feel safe.***

If we are in our threat system, we will still not feel calm and soothed just because there is no threat. Instead, we stay on alert ready for when the threat does appear. To feel safe and soothed we need to receive signals of safeness. These can be from outside of us, such as a good friend ringing us when we were feeling alone, or from inside of us, for example recalling memories of when we felt safe or doing a compassionate mind practice.

24. ***Just being uncertain of safeness is enough to start our threat system going.***

If what makes us feel safe starts to disappear, or we feel less certain it will be there when we need it, then our threat system starts to be released, like letting go of a dog that is eager to run.

25. ***If you feel 'anxious for no reason' look for a lack of safeness rather than presence of threat.***

We can sometimes look in the wrong place when we feel anxious. It may be that there is no threat, rather it is that we cannot detect the safeness we need to feel settled.

26. ***There is no such thing as 'too much safeness'.***

We can worry that if we surround ourselves or our baby with safeness then we (or our baby) will become unable to deal with struggles when they arise. If we are feeling worried or anxious about this, then this is our threat system that is in charge rather than our safeness system. Within our safeness system is courage and a willingness to learn new skills and engage with what scares us to build our confidence. As our confidence and skills build, we feel safer in the world. So, our safeness system enables us to feel more confident rather than less.

27. ***If we, or our baby, feel scared and anxious, check there is a secure base and a safe haven.***

A secure base is an external relationship, i.e. a person, or even the thought of a person, who gives us confidence to be able to do difficult things. This could be within us too in the form of our compassionate self or compassionate other. A safe haven is the person we can come back to when we get upset or overwhelmed who helps to calm us back down and regulate us. Again, this could be inside or outside of us. If these are absent, then we can get scared and anxious even when there is no actual threat. Rather we have lost our signals of safeness.

28. ***Life is full of suffering, but this is what our compassionate mind is here to help us with.***

We are wired to want to avoid suffering and find safeness. However, the very nature of being alive, and of having both an old and a new brain, means that we will encounter a lot of suffering; we know that we will decay and die, as will our loved ones, we are able to criticise ourselves and be criticised by others, we are wired to fear being cast out because for most of our human life this would most likely have meant death. Railing against suffering causes more suffering. Instead, if we can develop a way of knowing that no matter what happens to us in life, we will get through it, or be able to deal with it, or get up eventually after each and every knock down. Then that in itself gives us an immense sense of safeness. This is what the compassionate mind approach is all about.

My reminders:

Add here any phrases, pictures, diagrams, etc., that you have found help you to remember particular things about the compassionate mind approach. You might also want to add any 'reminders' from your baby and from your partner.

Module 63: My notes from throughout the book

(You might want to include diagrams, drawings, pictures, and so on – whatever you would find helpful. You might want to stick in more pages if you need to):

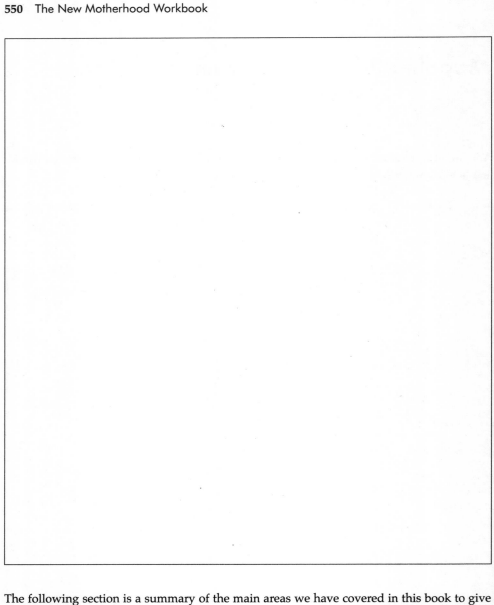

The following section is a summary of the main areas we have covered in this book to give an overall sense of the journey or 'story' of developing and using our compassionate mind in motherhood.

Module 64: Compassionate mind approach to new motherhood in a nutshell

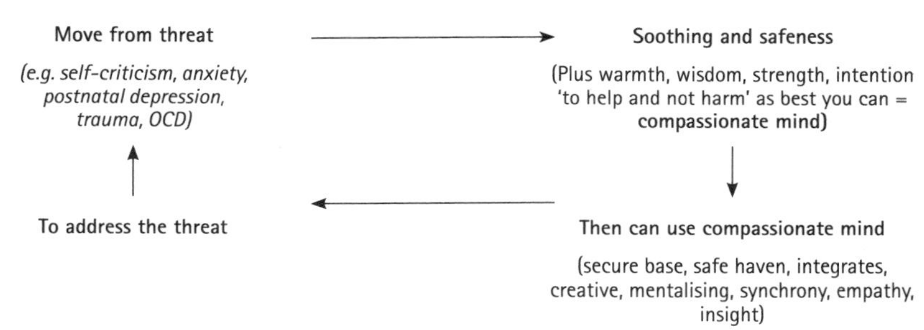

<table>
<tr><th colspan="3">Overview</th></tr>
<tr><th>'It's complicated'</th><th>'It's not your fault'</th><th>'Switch systems'</th></tr>
<tr><td>Perinatal period shaped by millions of years of evolution.

Much of which we aren't aware of but will influence us.</td><td>We have a mind evolved to seek safeness and to be alarmed by the risk of being cast out of the group or forgotten.

Our human mind is able to criticise and shame ourselves, and others, when we fear disconnection.

But criticism and shame create a narrow-focused pattern of threat in our mind and body.

It makes it hard for us to solve problems, and to get out of states of anxiety, depression or anger.

But this is not our fault.</td><td>We are wired to be highly responsive to signals of safeness, compassion, warmth, kindness.

This regulates threat, changing the way our mind and body function enabling:

Open attention, creative solutions, integrating new information, rest and digest, healing, reducing inflammation.

We can learn to deliberately switch into this pattern when we find ourselves in threat.

Then we carry on with what we were doing: problem solving; caring for baby; relating to others; relating to ourselves; etc., but from a pattern of safeness and compassion, rather than threat.</td></tr>
<tr><td colspan="3">But this is not our fault</td></tr>
</table>

'It's complicated' (Overview in more detail)

1. **Evolved brain:**
   i) Old brain with motives, emotions, behaviours
   ii) 'Human' new brain – reasoning, understands minds of others, conscious of consciousness (mindfulness)

Three emotion regulation systems:

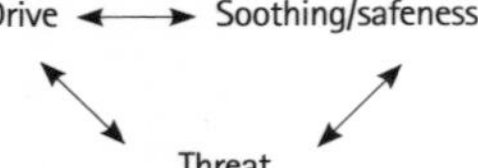

2. **Experiences**

   e.g. if brought up by different family such as next-door neighbours

Own experiences of being a child (for example, attachment strategies, memories, emotional conditioning/body memories, e.g. to oxytocin)

What learned about others (especially external fears) *e.g. 'People abandon you'*

What we have learned about ourselves in relation to others (especially internal fears) *e.g. 'I am unlovable', 'my emotions are harmful to others'.*

'It's not your fault' (Overview in more detail)

e.g. Tricky brain – old and new brain gets caught in loops.

Respond to our own face and voice as if outside of us. Has neurophysiological impact on us.

Ability to self-criticise.

Yearning for connection.

Fast track to threat.

We develop safety strategies to try to prevent further harm coming to us.

(e.g. to stop people hurting me I will keep them at a distance)

But these can have unintended consequences

(now I am alone. This is hard for humans especially when we have a new baby)

These are not our fault

(create different way forward through our compassionate mind)

= Formulation:

Back-ground	Fears	Safety Strategies	Unintended Conse-quences

'Switch systems' (Overview in more detail)

Need to be able to:

1. **Pause**
2. **Notice the 'pattern' or 'system' we are in.**
3. **Choose whether to change it.**

To change 'pattern' – 'Five stepping stones from threat to soothing':

Soothing breathing rhythm

1. **Posture**
2. **Breath**
3. **Mindfulness**
   'Body like a mountain, breath like the wind, mind like the sky.'
4. **Warm, kind face**
5. **Warm, kind voice**

Compassionate mind:

First engaging with the suffering.

Second – movement/action – doing something to alleviate and prevent the suffering.

Qualities:

1. **Strength** (body + 'benevolent authority'
2. **Courage**
3. **Wisdom** (evolution, experiences, 'not your fault', our 'intuitive wisdom')
4. **Motivation** ('heartfelt wish', intention, to help and not harm, to alleviate and prevent suffering)

3. Genetics *(e.g. temperament)* and Epigenetics (experiences can turn genes on and off) 4. **Evolved perinatal changes** *e.g. brain changes, hormonal, body.* Increased need for help from others/mother? 5. **Perinatal experiences** *e.g. pregnancy, birth, support, environment – which parenting algorithm triggered?* **6. Baby** *e.g. temperament, premature, unwell*		**Can train compassion, which changes the brain** (compassionate mind training): **Practice three flows – to others, from others, to selves:** **Practices** *e.g. using all senses – touch, smell, etc.* Compassionate place Compassionate colour Compassionate image Compassionate self Compassionate letter-writing Compassionate attention Compassionate behaviour Compassionate thinking Body, e.g. dance, yoga, martial art, singing Creating secure base and safe haven within ourselves, for us and for our baby. **Secure base** – facilitates exploration, learning new skills, builds confidence, brings joy, safeness **Safe haven** – provides soothing and regulation of threat system when become scared, angry, overwhelmed, dysregulated. This helps form foundation of **secure attachment**, for ourselves and baby. We need the skills of **mentalisation** (understanding that others have a separate mind to our own) and **synchrony** (adjusting our responses to those of another, e.g. our baby) – creating the relational 'dance'. These build the ability of our child to mentalise and build affiliative relationships with others **– it builds the compassionate mind of our child.** **These skills require safeness and compassionate mind, but also build and strengthen our own compassionate mind – a positive upward spiral.**

What would you add to this summary of the story or journey of developing a compassionate mind to new motherhood?

____

____

____

____

____

Module 65: Final words

What would your compassionate mind say to you about reaching this place in the workbook?

What would you like to say to your compassionate mind as you reach this point in your journey with them (which may be still in the early stages of learning and training)?

Thank you for taking this journey through this book.

Index

Note: page numbers in **bold** refer to diagrams.